CW00621175

FAMILY DOCTOR GUIDES

BMA

Asthma

Dr John Rees

Series editor: Dr Tony Smith

Dr Rees is a Senior Lecturer in Medicine and Consultant Physician at Guy's and Lewisham Hospitals.

EQUATION

Published by Equation in association with the British Medical Association

First published 1988

British Library Cataloguing in Publication Data

Rees, John, *1949-*
Asthma.
1. Man. Bronchi. Asthma
I. Title   II. Series
616.2'38

ISBN 1-85336-049-X

Picture acknowledgements

Wellcome Institute Library, London: p. 13; John Rae: pp. 23, 27,
51; Asthma Research Council: pp. 35, 65; Guy's Hospital Allergy
Clinic: p. 41; David Woodroffe: diagrams; Derek Marriott: cartoons.

Titles in the series:

Confusion in Old Age
Gallstones and Liver Problems
Arthritis
Asthma
Children's Health 1–5
Strokes and their Prevention

Equation, Wellingborough, Northamptonshire NN8 2RQ, England

Typeset by Columns of Reading
Printed and bound in Great Britain by The Bath Press, Avon

10 9 8 7 6 5 4 3 2 1

Contents

1 Introduction

Asthma is a very common condition that affects around 1 in 10 people. Although it usually begins in childhood, asthma can start at any age. There is a great range in the severity of asthma but in most cases it is a fairly mild problem easily controlled by simple treatment. The treatments for asthma are generally very effective and when used properly have very few side effects. What asthmatics need is to understand the common problems of asthma, and to know how to deal with them with drugs or by other means.

Asthma is a very variable disease and its symptoms are always changing. Asthmatics themselves are in the best position to evaluate these changes, sometimes with the help of measurements at home and with the advice of their doctors. So the answer to coping with the day to day problems of asthma is for asthmatics to be active in the management of their own disease and parents in the management of their children's.

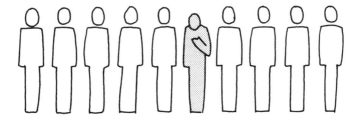

Help but not cure

Many things can be done to reduce problems with asthma but in most cases there is no cure. Some asthmatics have just one specific allergy which can be avoided, others have their problems brought on as a side effect of some other treatment. In these cases it may be possible to get rid of the asthma by removing the trigger but these cases are in the minority. Most people have many triggers for their asthma, or factors such as pollens or dust which are not really avoidable, or they may have no obvious triggers at all, and for them treatment will be necessary to suppress the disease.

7

Most asthma is easily controlled but a few sufferers have severe problems from their disease and in the United Kingdom there are nearly 2000 deaths from asthma every year. Only about 50 of these deaths occur in asthmatics under the age of 15, that is, one out of more than 20 000 asthmatics. Studies of these severe cases show that usually the patient or the doctor has failed to realise the severity of the attack and too little treatment has been given.

Understanding helps

Most people find it more satisfactory to take drugs when they understand the reasons for the treatment and, in general terms, how it is helping them. This brings us back again to education of asthmatic people and their families. This is the aim of many chest physicians and general practitioners today, to decrease the problems with asthma by increasing the understanding and involvement of their patients. It is also the aim of this book, and of local branches of the Friends of the Asthma Society.

2 What is asthma?

This may sound a very easy question to answer. We can all recognise asthma in a child who develops wheezing from contact with grass pollen or dust around the house or from exercise. This comes from narrowing of the air passages (airways) in the lungs. But there are problems with such a definition in many cases and experts have argued long and hard about the precise way in which asthma should be defined. It is difficult to diagnose in small babies, whose airways are so small that wheezing can be very easily provoked, and in older patients whose cigarette smoking has led to chronic bronchitis and emphysema that cause narrowing of the airways which cannot be improved by time or treatment. Most definitions of asthma run something like:

Asthma is a condition in which there is widespread narrowing of airways in the lungs which changes in severity over short periods of time spontaneously or with treatment.

In practical terms this means that there is breathlessness and wheezing which is worse sometimes than others. This sounds satisfactory until you begin to ask questions such as, 'How much narrowing of the airways?' and 'How much change does there need to be?' The definition works well for typical cases but tends to fray at the edges a little when it is stretched. This has led to some confusion for patients who may be told that they have asthma by one doctor but not by another.

Case history — Julia

Julia is 4. Her mother had noticed that she had been getting disturbed nights with coughing and some wheezing. This had been happening more and more often. It had started when she was 3 years old as occasional coughing during the night. After one bout lasting four consecutive nights Julia was taken to her general practitioner, who diagnosed an acute attack of bronchitis and gave her a course of antibiotics. The next coughing episode occurred six weeks later with some wheezing as well. On this occasion it was called wheezy bronchitis and slowly settled down with another course of antibiotics. There were three more similar episodes over the next five months. On the last occasion a locum doctor diagnosed the attacks as asthma not wheezy bronchitis and began treatment for asthma rather than giving antibiotics, with good results. Since this time Julia has been taking bronchodilators at the start of any similar episodes and has been nearly free of any trouble.

Comment

Asthma, as we will see later, often shows up in problems during the night, and coughing is a common symptom. It is likely that the symptoms which Julia had were asthma from the start. There was a feeling among some doctors that the term asthma would upset parents and that the term wheezy bronchitis was preferable. Unfortunately the common result of this is that unsuitable treatment is then given: antibiotics instead of asthma medications. It seems strange to try to conceal the identity of an illness which nearly always responds well to treatment and when this treatment depends upon the cooperation and understanding of the parents.

With children under about 18 months it is very difficult to be sure about the diagnosis of asthma because occasional bouts of wheezing are common with mild viral infections and most of the children who have these bouts do not go on to have asthma. By Julia's age, however, this is not a problem, and recurrent bouts of waking at night with cough and breathlessness are very likely to be asthma.

We will see later that the way to treat such a condition might be to deal with symptoms as they arise, as Julia's locum doctor did, or to give regular treatment to stop the attacks coming on.

Case history — George

Aged 65, George has smoked 25 cigarettes a day since the age of 15. Over the past 10 years he has become increasingly short of breath and this had reached the point where he had to stop once while going up the flight of stairs to his bedroom. This made him go to see his doctor who referred him to the local chest clinic. There he had some breathing tests and was given some inhalers to see if the results of his breathing tests improved. He saw three different doctors on his two visits to the clinic and one visit to the respiratory function laboratory for his breathing tests. The first doctor told him the problem was bronchitis, the second called it chronic obstructive airways disease and the third said it was asthma. George was given some inhalers and a short course of tablets which led to some improvement in his walking, but he was left confused about the real problem and whether or not he had asthma.

Comment

Older smokers who have narrowing of the airways can present a problem for the doctor in deciding whether they have asthma or chronic bronchitis and emphysema from their cigarette smoking. This cigarette smoking related condition has been given a large number of names, chronic obstructive airways disease is one of the more common ones. In practice it makes little difference what label is used though different names confuse the patient. If there is narrowing of the airways, as there would be if it was chronic asthma or if it was the result of damage from cigarette smoking, the treatment is to try to widen the airways and reverse the narrowing process with inhalers and tablets. The same treatment will be used whatever label is given in this case and most doctors will tend to use the term asthma if they find that the response to these treatments is good but tend towards chronic bronchitis and emphysema if the response is poor. As long as the right treatment is given the label does not matter.

Diagnosis is not always easy

I hope these two examples have shown that the diagnosis of asthma is not always quite as easy as you might think. The importance of making the diagnosis is to make sure that the right action is taken, which means identifying the factors that trigger off asthma and starting suitable treatment.

The history of asthma

Asthma has been recognised for over 2000 years but for a long time there was confusion between asthma and other causes of breathlessness. The word asthma comes from a Greek word meaning panting. Hippocrates, the great Greek physician, who lived from 460 to 370 BC on the island of Kos and is often regarded as the father of medicine, used the term asthma for any shortness of breath. Hippocrates recommended that asthmatics should avoid anger and shouting, which can certainly make asthma worse but are not always so easily avoided.

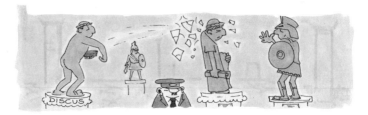

The 16th century

In the 16th century asthma began to be properly recognised, especially by the English physician Thomas Willis, although its nervous aspects were inappropriately emphasised. The first major book on the subject was called *A Treatise of the Asthma* and was written by Sir John Floyer and published in 1698. Floyer himself had asthma from childhood but it certainly did not shorten his life since he lived to be 85. Floyer recognised many of the features of asthma, such as the worsening at night, occupational asthma, and triggering by exercise and tobacco smoke. He noted that 'all Asthmatics, being angry or sad, do fall into Fits oftener than when they are cheerful'. Treatment was not so readily available at this time; some effective herbal remedies had been used for hundreds of years in the Far East, but were not known to Floyer.

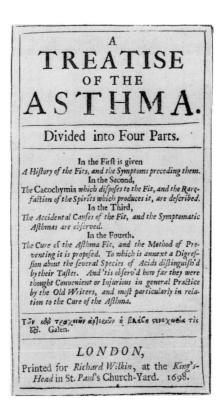

The 19th and 20th centuries

In the late 19th and early 20th centuries asthma came to be wrongly regarded as a trivial condition. Oliver Wendell Holmes, the American author and doctor, described it as a 'slight ailment which prolongs longevity'. Over the past 50 years great efforts have been made to improve the treatment of asthma and our understanding of the condition. This has led to the production of drugs which are increasingly effective and act almost exclusively on the airways, producing few side effects. The increase in interest and research into asthma has led to a better understanding of what it is but has not led to any real cure. Perhaps continued research will allow us to get rid of the problem but for the time being we need to continue to suppress the symptoms with the treatments that we have.

Normal lungs

Many factors lead to the narrowing of the airways in asthma, and even in between attacks — when there are no symptoms and measurements such as the peak flow rate are normal — the airways are not normal. In order to understand what is going wrong in the lungs in asthma we first need to understand a little about the normal structure and function of the lungs.

The most obvious function of the lungs is that of taking in oxygen from the air into the blood and getting rid of the waste gas carbon dioxide. In order to do this air has to be brought very close to the blood and this happens in tiny air sacs called alveoli. These are like tiny bubbles with thin blood vessels running in the walls of the bubbles. These alveoli are the end of an extensive branching structure which starts with the main airway into the lung, the trachea.

The airways

The entrance to the trachea can be closed to stop food or other objects entering the lungs by the epiglottis, which hangs over the entrance, and by the vocal cords, which can come together across the trachea like two shutters. The trachea is about two centimetres in diameter and runs for 10 centimetres before it divides up into the left and right main bronchi which supply the two lungs. In children, of course, all the airways are

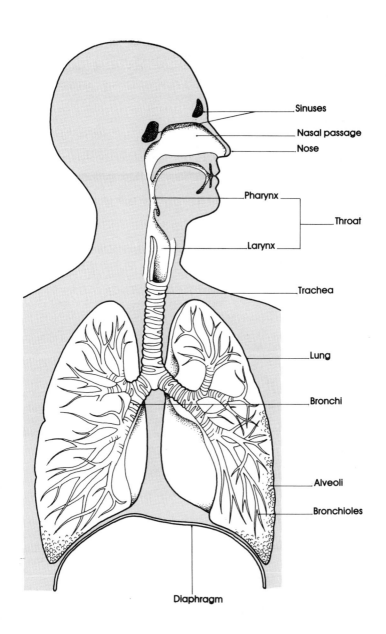

Sinuses

Nasal passage

Nose

Pharynx

Larynx

Throat

Trachea

Lung

Bronchi

Alveoli

Bronchioles

Diaphragm

smaller. The trachea is only half a centimetre wide in an infant and one centimetre by the age of 7. The bronchi branch many times to form the tiny tubes which supply the alveoli. For alveoli near the middle of the lung there will be about 10 branches while for those at the outside of the lung there may be 25. There are great numbers of small airways so that many may be narrowed by disease or lost before any symptoms or signs of the fact become apparent.

The alveoli

The alveoli are each about a quarter of a millimetre in diameter and there are about 300 million of them in the lungs. The total surface area of the alveoli available for the transfer of oxygen and carbon dioxide is about the size of a tennis court.

The circulation of the blood

Blood from the veins drains into the right side of the heart and is then pumped through the lungs by way of the tiny vessels in the walls of the alveoli. There it picks up oxygen and gets rid of carbon dioxide before returning to the left side of the heart to be pumped out to all the tissues in the body through the arteries.

Breathing in and out

Air comes in and out of the lungs through the pumping action of muscles. Even if we just sit still doing nothing 500 litres of air is breathed in and out every hour. The muscles in the diaphragm and the rib cage enlarge the chest, and air flows into the lungs through the trachea and all its branches. Breathing out (or expiration) is usually a passive process — that is, the muscles just relax and the lungs go down like a balloon deflating. However, the lungs do not get rid of all their air; a litre or two remains no matter how hard you try to breathe out.

Breathing takes effort

A little work is entailed in breathing in for all of us but there are two things that make this work much harder: the first is stiffness of the lungs, which makes them harder to expand and the second is narrowing of the air passages, which means that more effort has to be put in to pulling the air through them and air may have to be pushed out actively. Breathing through a narrow tube is very hard work and is just what the asthmatic has to do in a bad attack.

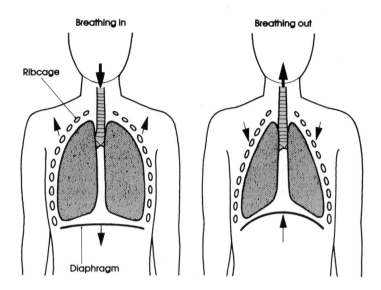

Ribcage

Diaphragm

The movement of the ribs and diaphragm lead to expansion and contraction of the lungs.

In asthma

When the air passages narrow, as in asthma, the lung seems to try to keep the air passages as large as possible by keeping more air in the lungs, this is called overinflation. It means that there is less room to take more air in with each breath, and breathing in becomes difficult while breathing out is limited by the narrow airways. Patients with acute attacks of asthma usually find it most comfortable to sit up so that their main muscle of respiration, the diaphragm, works best and they even use extra muscles in the neck to help their breathing.

The structure of the airways

The large airways such as the trachea have a stiff wall, which contains cartilage, the same substance as supports your nose and your ears. This makes these large airways less likely to narrow in asthma. All the airways are covered in an epithelium, which is like a thin skin, and on the top of this skin are tiny hairs called cilia which are constantly in motion wafting up the lung secretions from the outer portions of the lungs to the large airways. Some cells in the epithelium called goblet cells are

17

active in making some of these secretions. Underneath the epithelial layer there is a loose mass of tissue called connective tissue in which there are two important structures, the bronchial glands and the smooth muscle.

The bronchial glands   These have little tubes opening on to the inner surface of the airway and through these they are able to pour secretions of mucus into the airway where again it is wafted up to the larger airways and then coughed up or swallowed. In asthma the glands may produce mucus which is abnormally sticky and adds to the narrowing of the airways. In the lungs of those patients who do die of asthma the most remarkable feature is the fact that most of the air passages are blocked by sticky plugs of mucus.

Smooth muscle   Smooth muscle in the wall is able to narrow the airways if it contracts. The muscle is under the control of nerves, of substances circulating in the blood, and of local influences such as chemicals released from cells in the wall of the airway. There are several nerve supplies in the lungs, but the supply to the muscle which has been best studied runs in the vagus nerve. There are nerve endings in the airways like the nerves in the skin that respond to pain. When these are stimulated by a signal such as dust or cigarette smoke they send a message up to the brain. In the skin this would lead to the sensation of pain but in the lungs it leads to a signal being sent back down to the lungs through the vagus nerve which causes the muscle to contract and narrow the airways.

The airways in asthma

There are three main factors involved in the narrowing of the airways in asthma. These are:

- Contraction of the smooth muscle;
- Swelling of the connective tissue in the wall;
- Sticky mucus in the air passage.

Researchers have paid much attention to contraction of the smooth muscle (bronchoconstriction) in asthma. It is certainly important but so is swelling of the wall. This is a sign of inflammation in the wall of the airway and is similar to the inflammatory swelling which develops when the skin is burned or grazed. It is composed of fluid and of cells which release substances that attract other cells; this causes more swelling and leads to contraction of the muscle. Research has shown that this inflammation remains to some degree in the walls of asthmatics even when they are free of any problems and even when the disease has not given any trouble for 6 to 12 months. These cells are still sitting in the airway wall waiting for the right stimulus to be activated again and spark off the changes which lead to an attack of asthma.

Mast cells

Many sorts of inflammatory cells in the wall of the airway are important in asthma. Those which have been best studied are the mast cells. These contain little packages which they can release if they are triggered in the right way, for instance by a pollen grain in somebody with the right allergy. These little packages contain highly active substances which cause the muscle to contract, produce swelling of the wall of the airway, and attract more inflammatory cells to the area, so increasing the inflammation and the response to any further stimulus.

Effect of drugs

The drugs used for asthma work mainly on these two abnormalities — the smooth muscle contraction and the swelling of the airways. The persistent inflammation is probably what keeps an asthmatic person at risk of further attacks and it needs prolonged regular treatment to bring it under control. Left unchecked it may be responsible for further changes in the airways that cause scarring and eventually limit the possibility of reversing the narrowing of the airways. In this way the persistence of inflammation may change asthma from an intermittent, reversible obstruction to a fixed narrowing which drug treatment can no longer help.

3 Who gets asthma?

Asthma is a common condition throughout the world and there is evidence to suggest that it is getting more common in countries such as the United Kingdom, United States, Australia, and Scandinavia. There is, however, a lot of geographical variation and in some communities there is very little asthma indeed. In the Gambia and among Eskimos asthma is uncommon. Studies in villagers in the highlands of New Guinea 20 years ago showed very little asthma but later studies have shown that even in this primitive rural community asthma is on the increase.

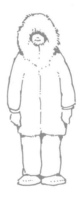

How common is asthma?

In most westernised countries asthma is the commonest important disease in children. Studies in the UK suggest that at around the age of 7 years, 11 to 12% of children will be affected by asthma in any one year. This is more than one in 10 children and one in every five children will have shown features of asthma at some stage by the time they reach the age of 10. Boys are affected more commonly than girls. The ratio is around two boys to one girl at the age of 7 but it begins to even out above this age since boys are more likely to lose their asthma as they get older.

In adults the exact amount of asthma is a little difficult to be sure of owing to problems with the precise definition of asthma mentioned in the last chapter. In questionnaire studies in the UK and USA around 30% of adults said they had wheezing of the chest. Not all of these will actually have asthma and the real rate is probably nearly 6% (one in 16) of adults with asthma symptoms in any one year.

Asthma in families

Asthma has a strong tendency to run in families. In 1946 the population of the island of Tristan da Cunha in the Atlantic Ocean was studied, and nearly one half of the inhabitants were found to have asthma. This was traced back to three asthmatic women who were among the original 15 settlers on the island and it shows the strong genetic element in the inheritance of asthma. But there is no simple genetic explanation for the inheritance.

Two factors

It is possible that there are two separate tendencies being inherited, a tendency to form antibodies against common substances such as pollen or house dust, and a tendency for the airways to narrow easily. When these two are combined and the environment produces the right stimuli then asthma occurs. The body produces these substances called antibodies when it meets a new substance. They are generally protective and help in resisting infections but in some circumstances, such as asthma, the antibodies themselves may produce harmful reactions.

Atopy

The tendency to form these sorts of antibodies is known as atopy and occurs in one in three people. It can be shown by skin tests which react to pollen, house dust mite, cat fur, and the like (p. 41). Atopy is related to two other conditions that run in the same families as asthma: hay fever and childhood eczema; some asthmatics suffer from these as well as asthma.

The environment

Genes are certainly not the only determinant of asthma; the environment is also important. This has been seen with the changing rates of asthma among the Tokelau islanders who moved to mainland New Zealand and among those who have moved from the Indian subcontinent to the UK. Xhosa children in rural Transkei in southern Africa rarely have asthma but the rate of asthma increases 30 times if they move to live in urban Cape Town. The importance of other factors is also indicated by studies of twins since in an identical pair of twins when one is asthmatic the other commonly but not invariably also has the condition.

Inheritance

Children of an asthmatic parent have their chances of developing asthma increased 20 times but the chances depend on the severity of the parent's asthma. If one parent has asthma the child will have asthmatic symptoms in around 25% of cases (one in four) while if both parents have asthma the chances of the child having problems is around 40% (two in five). Some studies have suggested that the chances of children developing asthma are reduced by breast feeding. To be effective, this probably needs to be strict breast feeding right from the start and even though there is considerable disagreement about the findings it seems a sensible course for asthmatic parents to follow if possible.

Types of asthma

Extrinsic asthma

There are two broad types of asthma and the two follow rather different patterns. There is the type of asthma that comes on in childhood. This is often related to hay fever and eczema in the child or in other members of the family. In this form of asthma there are usually obvious factors which bring on attacks, such as house dust, pollens or animals fur; this can usually be confirmed by skin prick tests. Infections such as colds, emotion, and exercise often bring on attacks. Because of all these outside influences this is often called *extrinsic asthma*. In general there is a lot of variability in the amount of airway narrowing but response to treatment is very good.

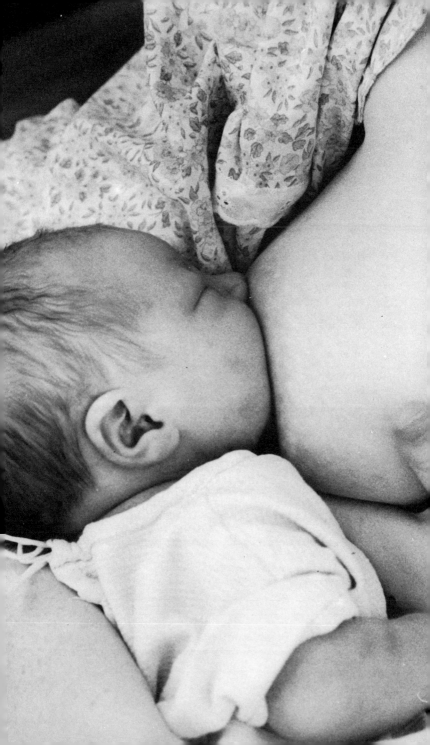

Intrinsic asthma

The other sort of asthma is called *intrinsic asthma* and is the sort that usually comes on in adult life. The asthmatic episodes are often brought on by upper respiratory infections, colds, and bronchitis, but other triggers are not usually so evident and skin tests are negative. The narrowing of the airways tends to be less easily reversible with treatment and these patients often have persistent symptoms.

These are just broad groups and many asthmatics may fall somewhere in between these types. In other types such as occupational asthma, there may be specific triggers which are not related to other sensitivities.

Asthma and other illnesses

People often suffer hay fever as well as asthma, particularly the extrinsic form. More than half of extrinsic asthmatics but only one in every 15 intrinsic asthmatics have hay fever. The other condition linked to atopy, childhood eczema, is found in about one third of asthmatics.

Bronchitis and emphysema

The first chapter mentioned the confusion between asthma and chronic bronchitis and emphysema produced by cigarette smoking. Asthma in adults is often persistent and difficult to reverse with treatment rather like chronic bronchitis and emphysema. The two conditions of chronic bronchitis and emphysema are nearly always found together and it is often rather difficult in life to tell how much of each a patient is suffering from. In chronic bronchitis the mucus glands (p. 18) enlarge and secrete excess mucus which is coughed up most days as sputum. In emphysema there is a breadkown in the walls of the alveoli (p. 16). Both conditions are related to narrowing of the airways in the lung. Asthma may occur with these other conditions, and asthmatic patients may well be at greater risk of these complications of smoking.

> **Inhalation of all forms of tobacco smoke is certainly a bad influence on asthma and should be avoided.**

Asthmatics should never smoke themselves and should try to avoid other people's smoke, so-called passive smoking. Children brought up in a home where parents smoke are more likely to have chest infections, and parents of asthmatic children have a particular responsibility not to smoke.

Pregnancy

Many other medical conditions have some relation to the control of asthma. Pregnancy and the menstrual cycle can also cause changes in asthma (p. 52).

Overweight

Obesity increases the work that the lungs have to do and should be avoided. The question of exercise and asthma is discussed further on page 46 but it is certainly wise to stay as fit as possible to ease the work of the lungs. For most asthmatics this is not a great problem although it may mean taking some medication before bouts of exercise. Even for those who are quite restricted by their asthma limited forms of exercise and careful control of the diet are still possible.

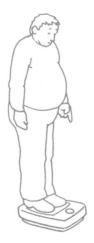

Other disorders

Many drugs can affect control of asthma (p. 48), forms of indigestion in which acid comes up from the stomach into the oesophagus may provoke attacks (p. 52), and changes in the behaviour of the thyroid gland may affect asthma control.

4 The natural course of asthma

Most parents are anxious to know whether their child will grow out of asthma, and several studies have provided this information, particularly a study from Melbourne in Australia which has followed up for over 20 years 200 children who were wheezing at the age of 7. Most children who are going to have asthma will have shown some sign of the trouble by this age. The natural course of asthma which comes on in adult life has not been so closely studied and nobody has managed to follow asthmatics right through their life to see the full pattern of the disease.

Growing out of asthma

Many children who have bouts of wheezing with infections in the first few years of life will not go on to have serious problems with their asthma. Three quarters of these children have no problems with asthma by the time they reach the age of 10. The study of 7 year olds in Melbourne has shown that in general the outlook is related to the amount of trouble the child is having with asthma.

Sometimes asthma goes

At the age of 7 three quarters of children with asthma have fairly mild problems, 20% have persistent symptoms which need continuous treatment, and 5% have severe problems.

Of children whose asthma is very mild or just consists of occasional wheezing nearly three quarters will be free of asthma seven years later at the age of 14. However, only 20% of those with a lot of problems at the age of 7 will lose their asthma over the next seven years. Boys have a better outlook than girls in these early years; although more develop asthma initially they are more likely to grow out of it. Even if asthma does not go away completely it tends to improve during puberty in most children.

But sometimes it recurs

Unfortunately, even if asthma goes away as children grow up there is no guarantee that it will stay away. One third of the children who had lost their asthma in the Australian study had problems again by the time they got into their 20s. It seems that the tendency to develop asthma is still in the background waiting to be given the right circumstances to show itself again. This has important implications for such children. They should avoid circumstances which are likely to provoke problems. Certainly they should not smoke and it seems wise to avoid prolonged contact with common allergens as much as possible. This will mean keeping dust down, and avoiding feather bedding and furry pets even when the asthma seems to have settled.

Children's pets may make asthma worse.

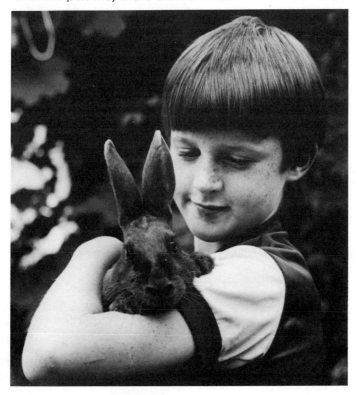

The outlook in adults

Once asthma comes on in adult life it seems to be much less likely to improve spontaneously. In adults asthma follows various patterns. Sometimes it is similar to that seen in childhood with a great deal of variability and good response to treatment. In other people it is more persistent; treatment has an effect but does not always return the situation to normal and needs to be used continuously.

Reversing damage is difficult

For many asthmatic patients fully reversing the narrowing of their airways is much more difficult in adult life than when they are young. This seems to have something to do with how severe their asthma is in childhood. Troublesome disease in children seems to be more likely to go on to permanent narrowing of the airways. The big unanswered question is whether adequate treatment to control the asthma in the younger patients prevents the development of this irreversibility. This is not known but it is very likely to be true and provides another reason for vigorously trying to achieve good control of asthma throughout life.

Problems from asthma

Asthma is responsible for more absences from school than any other chronic disease. This is especially so when it is unrecognised or not being properly treated. At present two thirds of asthmatics miss some time from school because of their condition and half of these miss more than three weeks each year.

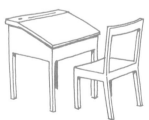

Work and social life

Persistent symptoms can limit the social and occupational life of adult asthmatics. If asthma is very severe it can put extra strain on the heart and may lead on to heart failure in a few people. Mostly the difficulties in adult life are to do with lack of mobility because of chronic problems and loss of time from work and home because of acute attacks.

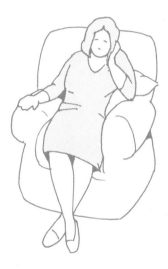

Hospital

Hospital admissions for asthma have increased over the past 10 years. There are many reasons for this. There is a greater tendency to admit asthmatics with acute attacks and some hospitals have started a self referral policy which means that asthmatic patients can get themselves admitted to hospital whenever they feel it is necessary. There also seems to have been a slight increase in the general severity of asthma as well as an increase in its frequency.

There is a variation through the year in the rate of hospital admissions for asthma and this is particularly noticeable in children. July, September, October, and November are the times of most frequent admission with the lowest rates in January and February. There are also variations through the day with most admissions occurring in the early morning hours as might be expected from the usual variation through the day in asthma severity (p. 36).

29

Case history — James

James started to have problems with asthma at the age of 4. These were intermittent for about two years but then throughout the rest of his school life asthma was a considerable problem. He was unable to play games at school. He went through all the available treatments for asthma during this time; some of them were effective but problems always recurred. Contact with animals and grass pollen gave him particular problems. He has never smoked. Although he was a little better in his late teens, he has had problems ever since. Now at the age of 55 he has persistent obstruction and can walk only 100 yards before he has to stop for a rest. Even with high doses of drugs in inhalers and tablets it is not possible to get further improvement and he needs continuous treatment to keep things as good as this.

Comment

If James had been seen first at the age of 55 and had been a smoker it would be tempting to put his trouble down to smoking. However, he has never smoked and from his problems it is clear that James has asthma. He had his early problems at a time when the available treatment was not so satisfactory although it used to give him some improvement. His asthma is now not nearly so reversible and he is quite disabled by his illness. Most doctors think that if adequate treatment had been available and he had been vigorously treated as a child his present condition might have been much better.

Deaths from asthma

Despite all the improvements in the treatment of asthma a depressing feature of the past 20 years has been the continuing death rate from asthma. Instead of declining this has been showing some signs of increasing. In the past there have been several temporary increases in the death rate from asthma; in the UK in the 1960s and in New Zealand in the early 1980s. Neither of these has been completely satisfactorily explained but they may have been because people relied too much on their usual bronchodilator treatment instead of seeking further help. At present there are nearly 2000 deaths from asthma each year in the UK. Nearly all these occur in adults — only 50 or less children die from asthma each year.

Don't underestimate the problem

Certainly all the investigations of deaths from asthma indicate that most of the problems result from doctors and patients underestimating the severity of an attack and either failing to seek help at all or not receiving suitable treatment. Very few if any of the deaths are caused by too much treatment or side effects of treatment. A careful analysis of a sample of deaths from asthma suggests that over half could have been prevented by better treatment, especially early treatment when the first signs of deterioration were apparent. All the studies come up with this same message: the main problem is not that the right treatments do not exist but that they do not get to the patient at the right time.

A careful study of the events preceding severe or fatal attacks of asthma shows that a few attacks are very sudden with a change from stable, trouble-free asthma to severe problems but that most attacks are preceded by days or weeks of the asthma gradually getting worse. There is usually plenty of time and warning to get in early and prevent the severe attack if the right action is taken.

Every asthmatic needs to work out with his or her doctor a plan of action to be followed when problems arise. After the first severe attack it may be too late so these plans need to be worked out before the troubles arise. They should be known to the patient and to those close to him. They will usually consist of changes in treatment or contact with a doctor or hospital.

Adjusting treatment or seeking help early enough is the most important factor in stopping severe attacks of asthma.

Changing the natural course of asthma

I have already mentioned the question of altering the natural course of asthma by proper early treatment to suppress the disease. This is most likely to act by reducing the inflammation in the airways in the lung. We will see later that the drugs most likely to do this are the suppressors of inflammation such as corticosteroids, sodium cromoglycate, and nedocromil. These drugs can reduce the reactions of the airways to all the various stimuli that lead to narrowing of the airways.

Avoid allergens

The other way to change the general reactions of the airways is to reduce the contact with factors which the asthmatic is allergic to. It can be easily done if there is just one factor but this is unusual except in the case of occupational asthma (p. 49). Even if there are lots of trigger factors it is worth reducing the general load on the airways. For example, if there are reactions to house dust mite, grass pollen, and cat fur it is worth avoiding cats and reducing house dust mite as much as possible. Over long periods of time this may help to reduce the responses of the airways to all sorts of other non-specific factors such as smoky and dusty atmospheres as well.

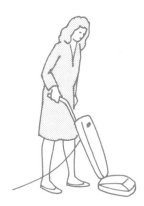

Desensitising

Another approach to reducing the responses to specific factors has been to try to reduce the allergic response by 'desensitising' the asthmatic patient. This requires a course of injections consisting of small amounts of the very substance which is causing the allergic response. This approach has been disappointing in the management of asthma and has some dangers. It is discussed further on page 79.

5 How to recognise asthma

The three main symptoms of asthma are shortness of breath, wheezing, and cough. None of these is unique to asthma. Wheezing is a whistling sound caused by vibration of the walls of an air passage like the reed in the mouthpiece of a toy trumpet. Although wheezing is the most characteristic of these features 30% of adults say that they have wheezing at some time and only about a quarter of these are likely to have asthma. Many people may have a little wheezing with a severe upper respiratory tract infection. Other conditions may cause wheezing, such as cystic fibrosis in children and chronic bronchitis and emphysema in adults.

Wheezing

In asthma there is widespread narrowing of many airways in the lung, but wheezing can also come from narrowing of one of the large airways such as the trachea (p. 14). Choking on a foreign body can partly block a large airway and produce wheezing. Adults can usually describe clearly what has happened but this may be more of a problem in children. In adults one of the main airways may be narrowed by a growth or some other condition and this may occasionally be confused with asthma.

Cough

When a cough is the main symptom asthma is particularly likely to go unrecognised. In children the cough is usually at its worst at night and with exercise. This may mean disturbed nights for children and for parents. Cough is less likely to be the only symptom in adults but this does sometimes happen. It may be difficult for doctors to find any evidence of narrowing of the airways in such patients. They may not fit into the conventional diagnosis of asthma but they do have irritability of the airways and they get better with conventional asthma treatment such as inhaled bronchodilators or inhaled corticosteroids.

In some ways this is similar to the irritating cough which non-asthmatic people sometimes get after a viral infection in the throat and upper airways. The virus damages the lining of the airways and makes it inflamed and irritable rather like an asthmatic's airways. In these circumstances we may all become mild asthmatics for a short time but in non-asthmatics the airway narrowing is limited and the damage is repaired within four to six weeks. There is something about asthmatic airways which makes them go on to narrow and which keeps the airway lining inflamed.

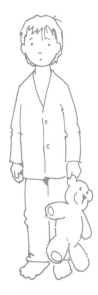

Cough is often worse at night.

Reversibility of airway narrowing

The definition of asthma on p. 9 mentions that the amount of narrowing of the airways varies. The usual way to go about confirming the diagnosis of asthma is to try to show this variability by reversing the narrowing with treatment. This is, of course, only possible if the patient has some narrowing at the time and it will not be appropriate for those who have occasional attacks and are completely back to normal when they go to see the doctor.

Assessment

Assessment of reversibility generally means making a measurement of the degree of narrowing and then repeating the measurements after giving some treatment to reverse it. This treatment will usually be a bronchodilator taken by inhaler. Salbutamol (Ventolin) is the one most often used. The measurement can be done in various ways as described on p. 53 but the simplest is to measure the peak flow rate. This means blowing out as hard as possible into a small meter. If the airways are narrowed then the speed the air can come out of the lungs is limited and when the salbutamol widens the airways the flow rate measurements increase.

In a simple assessment of reversibility this will mean three blows into a peak flow meter then two puffs of an inhaler followed by three more blows into the meter 15 to 20 minutes later. The doctor will be looking for a change of at least 15 to 20% in the measurement to be convinced that there is reversibility. If this size of change can be seen then there is little doubt about the diagnosis.

Measuring the peak flow rate using a portable meter. This is a good test of the effectiveness of treatment.

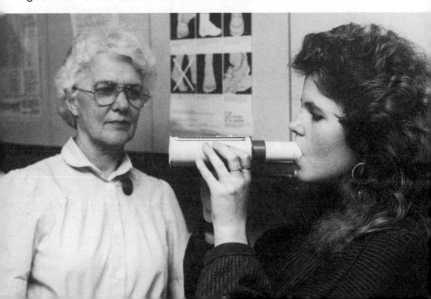

More severe narrowing

Sometimes the narrowing of the airways is not so easy to reverse, and larger doses or different drugs will be necessary. This will require more extensive testing using higher doses of the same inhaler or another inhaler such as ipratropium bromide. It may also require more complex measurement techniques to show that changes are occurring.

Steroids

In some circumstances, particularly in older patients with persistent problems, it may be necessary to give a course of oral corticosteroids for a week or two in order to look for reversibility. These tests of the effects of treatment on the narrowing of the airways not only help in the diagnosis of asthma but also give information about the improvement to be expected from treatment and the treatments which are most likely to be effective.

Measuring natural variability in asthma

If there is no problem with asthma and no narrowing of the airways when the patient sees the doctor then some other method has to be used to demonstrate the condition. One simple way is to look for the natural variation which usually occurs in asthma. When asthmatics record their peak flow rate throughout the day many of them show a characteristic pattern of producing their highest results in the afternoon and their lowest levels during the early hours of the morning. This is called diurnal variation of asthma or the 'morning dip'. The lowest point is usually at 3 or 4 in the morning, a time when many asthmatics wake up with wheezing if their asthma is not well controlled. Non-asthmatic people also have a diurnal variation in their peak flow rate but it is very small and barely noticeable.

Morning dipping

In order to look for morning dipping it is not necessary to wake up throughout the night to blow into the peak flow meter; measurements first thing in the morning on waking and in the evening will suffice. The patient takes home a peak flow meter and measures the best result two or three times a day for two weeks. If the morning results are on average 15% lower than the evening values then the diagnosis of asthma is confirmed.

Other patterns of asthma may be found by regular peak flow recording and this is an important way of investigating asthma thought to be related to work. Regular peak flow recording at home is also very important in the assessment of changes in treatment and in the day to day monitoring of the disease (p. 54).

The cause of the morning dipping in asthma is unknown. There have been many theories concerning the effects of sleep itself, cold air, hormones, daytime treatments running out and so on but none of them have really provided satisfactory explanations.

Provoking airway narrowing

An alternative to home peak flow recording to look for morning dipping is to see how easy it is to provoke asthma. There are three main ways of doing this, which are of increasing complexity. The simplest approach is by looking for the effects of exercise.

Exercise testing

Asthmatic patients often notice that they become wheezy with exercise and in tests 80 to 90% of asthmatics can be made to wheeze with exercise. Very complex apparatus can be used to monitor breathing during exercise but to demonstrate exercise-induced asthma only a simple test is necessary. This requires six minutes of vigorous exercise, which can be running around the outside of the surgery or up and down stairs. In normally healthy people the airways actually get a little wider during exercise; in asthmatics this may happen also but it is followed by a narrowing of the airways which is usually greatest about 5 to 10 minutes after exercise. Peak flow rate is measured before and after exercise. If it drops by more than 15% after exercise then the test is positive and the narrowing can be reversed by an inhaled bronchodilator.

Exercise testing is a safe test in asthma and can be performed at a general practitioner's surgery without complex equipment. Care is necessary with older patients who have heart disease.

The cause of the exercise-induced asthma is probably drying and cooling of the airways, and some laboratories use cold air, dry air, or mists of salty water instead of exercise tests.

Airway responsiveness to methacholine and histamine

The airways of asthmatic patients react to many substances much more quickly and more dramatically than the airways of non-asthmatics. Two substances are commonly used to show this increased responsiveness. They are histamine, which is a chemical released from inflammatory cells in the airways, or methacholine which stimulates the nerve endings in the walls of the airways. These substances are given in increasing amounts by inhalation until a drop in peak flow rate or some other measurement has occurred. Many normally healthy people can be made to wheeze with these substances but it needs much higher doses than those needed for asthmatics.

Over-responsive airways

These tests need to be carried out in hospital laboratories and they are not often necessary to diagnose asthma. One of the tests above — reversibility, morning dipping, or exercise testing — is usually enough. However, the use of histamine or methacholine brings out a very important concept in asthma, the state of over-responsiveness of the airways. Asthmatics' airways are 'twitchy'; they respond to tiny doses of these substances by narrowing. This twitchiness is probably a result of the inflammation in the walls, which increases the release of active compounds from the inflammatory cells and the ease with which the nerves can be stimulated.

The over-responsiveness means that the inflamed airways of asthmatics are likely to narrow in response to all sorts of stimuli — for example, exercise, cold air, or dusts — as well as to specific allergic stimuli such as pollen grains. This responsiveness can be seen in asthmatics even when the disease seems to have given no trouble for a year or more. The airways of people with hay fever have an intermediate level of responsiveness between those of normally healthy and asthmatic people. When asthmatics have infections or contact with substances they are allergic to the inflammation in the airways is increased and their over-responsiveness may be increased for days or weeks afterwards. Some drugs such as inhaled corticosteroids can reduce the responsiveness if taken regularly. Bronchodilator drugs will reduce or abolish the responses if used just before contact with a known trigger for asthma.

Case history — Jack

Jack is aged 45. He never had trouble with asthma until he was 40. Then he was diagnosed as having asthma brought on by chemicals called isocyanates at the factory where he worked making polyurethane foam. He had tried to go on working using various treatments to control his asthma but after two years he had left that job and gone to work in an office a mile or two from the factory. His asthma had gradually settled over the months after he left the firm and he had had no problems for the past two years. He went to see some of his old workmates at the factory one afternoon and went around the factory to see the changes which had been made.

The evening of his visit he had his first asthma attack for some years. Fortunately he still had a salbutamol inhaler at home and the attack settled with six puffs of salbutamol during the evening. Four times over the next week he woke up at night with wheezing around 3 am and had to take some salbutamol. He found that walking the three quarters of a mile to the office in the morning was making him short of breath. In the office he found that the smoke from a secretary's cigarettes was making him cough whenever he was in the room. All these problems gradually settled over two weeks and he was then back to normal again. He vows never to go back to the factory again.

Comment

Isocyanates are a common cause of occupational asthma but this might just as well have been some other trigger such as an animal. Jack's asthma had settled after leaving the work place but he still had the underlying tendency. When he was in contact with the trigger again he had an initial attack and this temporarily increased the responsiveness of his airways so that they reacted to cigarette smoke and to exercise, and his morning dipping returned. All these problems settled down again over two weeks because there was no further contact. A return to work in the factory would result in continued over-responsiveness so that all sorts of other triggers as well as the isocyanates themselves would affect Jack's asthma.

Specific tests

In the same way as the airways can be tested with the non-specific stimuli histamine and methacholine they can also be tested with suspected allergens. This would involve laboratory tests exposing someone thought to be allergic to pollen to a tiny amount of pollen extract or exposing Jack to a tiny amount of isocyanate. This may occasionally be necessary to confirm occupational asthma but is rarely necessary except as a research tool in other forms of asthma. It is only performed in suitable laboratories because severe asthma may be provoked if too large a dose is used and because asthmatic reactions may occur 6 or 8 hours after the test. These late asthmatic reactions are very mild and uncommon after exercise and are not seen with histamine or methacholine testing. They may well be more like real asthma than the narrowing occurring minutes after challenge but they are less predictable.

When allergies are being investigated it is usual to stick to simple procedures such as skin tests or blood tests rather than testing the airways.

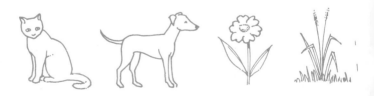

Skin tests

Skin tests are not really a diagnostic test for asthma but they can help in finding out which substances may provoke attacks. The finding of a positive skin test means that the patient has a specific type of antibody (IgE antibody) against that particular antigen. This shows that they are atopic (see p. 21) along with nearly 30% of the population. It does not necessarily show that this particular antigen is involved in the asthma. However, it would be unusual to find that an inhaled allergen was relevant to a patient's asthma when the skin test was negative.

The skin tests are performed by putting a little drop of the extract on to the forearm and then very gently pricking the skin underneath. This is a painless procedure which does not draw blood. If the test is positive an itchy lump appears on the skin within the next 20 minutes and then subsides over the next hour. The size of the lump is measured and 2 mm and over is a significant size. The only drugs that significantly affect the results are antihistamines. If a person is taking these for hay fever at the time the skin tests will be negative. The tiny amount of the extract used has no effect on the state of the asthma at the time.

Skin tests help identify substances that provoke attacks of asthma.

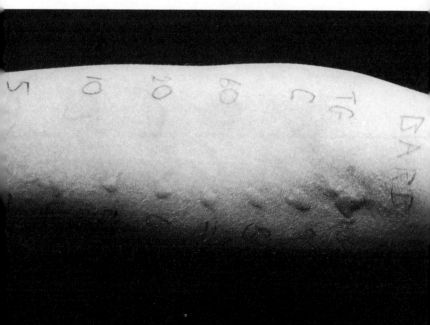

6 Triggers of asthma

Some asthmatics soon learn that there are factors which bring on their asthma and learn to avoid these as much as possible. The most obvious are usually substances which produce wheezing within minutes of being breathed in. If the culprit is an animal such as a cat then to a large extent this can be avoided. If the problem comes from substances which are widely distributed in the home or outdoor environment, such as house dust mites or pollen grains, then it is much more difficult to avoid them.

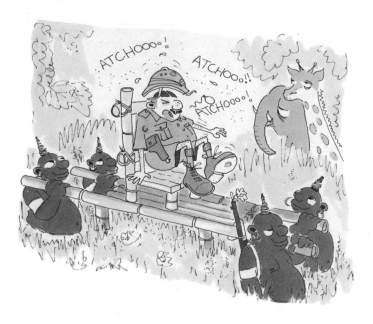

Most asthmatics have their asthma brought on by a number of different factors because they have over-responsiveness of the airways. These trigger factors are generally easier to identify in young asthmatics. Some triggers such as foods are more controversial and are more difficult to detect. In this chapter we will deal with the various factors that can provoke asthma and to some extent what can be done about them.

Infection

Infections of the upper respiratory tract; colds, influenza, sore throats and tracheitis are the factors which most often bring on acute attacks of asthma. Most of these infections are caused by viruses. These viruses can damage the lining of the airways, stripping off the delicate covering, exposing the nerve endings, and attracting inflammatory cells into the damaged area. We have seen that these changes are likely then to increase the tendency of the airways to narrow in response to all sorts of stimuli.

Virus infections in the first few years of life are particularly likely to produce wheezing because the smaller size of the infant's airway means that only a little narrowing is necessary to start causing trouble. These infections in infancy may be followed by recurrent bouts of wheezing but most of those who have these wheezy attacks in the first year of life do not go on to get asthma.

Antibiotics don't work

Because most of these infections are caused by viruses they are not affected by conventional antibiotics. Some of the infections are caused by bacteria and sometimes a viral infection may be complicated by a bacterial infection as well. Antibiotics may be used to treat the bacterial infection, but not without specific treatment of the asthma.

Asthmatic people who do have attacks brought on by infections are usually advised to have an influenza immunisation when it becomes available early each autumn. This will not guarantee a winter free of infections but it will reduce problems with some of the common viruses.

Allergens that are breathed in

Allergens are the tiny particles which can spark off an allergic asthmatic attack when they are breathed in by someone with asthma who already has specific antibodies. The allergen (or antigen) and the antibody combine on the surface of inflammatory cells such as mast cells and this reaction releases the little packets of mediators from the inside of the cell. The presence of the antibodies can be proved by positive skin prick tests (p. 41). If skin tests are positive it means that the antibodies are present but not necessarily that this allergen is involved in the particular patient's asthma.

There are three common sources of such allergens involved in asthma in the UK. These are:

- house dust mites
- pollens
- animals.

House dust mites

The house dust mite goes under the impressive name of *Dermatophagoides pteronyssinus* and when magnified is a fearsome looking creature. House dust mites are found all over the place; they feed on human skin scales that have been shed from the skin. Warm, humid environments suit house dust mites best and they are infrequent in cold, dry climates such as the higher mountains of Switzerland where asthmatics were often sent to clear up their asthma. The dust mites are found in all household dust but are particularly likely to accumulate where there are soft furnishings and dust traps. Fluffy toys which children like to cuddle in bed are an ideal resting place for them.

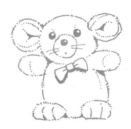

Even though it is too small to be seen with the naked eye the house dust mite itself is too big to be breathed in and cause a reaction inside the airways. The problem comes from particles of the mite droppings which are small enough to enter the airways and carry protein from the mite to which asthmatics respond with increased asthma.

House dust mites provide the commonest positive skin prick test in the UK. This tendency to form antibodies or atopy exists in up to 30% of the population. Among asthmatic children 80% have a positive skin prick test for house dust mite.

When asthmatics sensitive to the mite are put in environments free of it they get better but the mites are so numerous that it is impossible to remove them completely from the home. Attempts to reduce them substantially have been rather disappointing but it certainly seems worth trying to keep the contact down as much as possible. In practical terms this means the use of synthetic pillows and duvets instead of feather, and regular vacuum cleaning of mattresses, bedding, curtains, and carpets. Enclosing mattresses in polythene covers may also help and some new powders and solutions which kill the dust mites show some promise.

Reducing the allergic response by hyposensitisation is considered on page 79. Occasionally it may benefit asthmatics with severe house dust mite problems but in most cases the asthma is better controlled with simple drug treatment.

Pollens

The types of pollen responsible for asthma and hay fever depend on the local circumstances. Pollens are released at various times of the year but are most abundant in late spring and in summer. Pollen from some trees such as the silver birch and plane is released earlier in April and can be a particular problem in London from London plane trees. The symptoms of pollen sensitive asthma are often combined with eye and nose problems from hay fever.

Many grasses give problems, particularly Timothy grass, cocksfoot, and Bermuda grass. It is sensible to stay away from grass cutting and obvious high pollen areas but such widespread allergens cannot be completely avoided.

When problems occur in the late summer and early autumn they are likely to be caused by mould spores especially *Alternaria* which grows on grain and *Cladosporium* and *Aspergillus* which grow on rotting vegetation. The *Aspergillus* fungus produces a particular problem in some asthmatics as it grows in plugs of mucus within the airways and a strong allergic reaction permanently damages the surrounding airway wall. This condition is known as allergic bronchopulmonary aspergillosis, and it must be treated, usually with corticosteroids (p. 73).

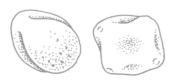

Animals

Almost all family pets can cause problems for asthmatics. Cats are most likely to give problems from allergens in the hair, skin scales, urine, and saliva. If one cat causes wheezing the same is likely to occur with most other cats. Some breeds such as Siamese seem to have their own individual allergens. Among dogs there seem to be more differences between species. Birds, rabbits, mice, other rodents, and horses can all cause trouble and in general asthmatics should avoid close contact with such animals.

Animals should always be kept out of an asthmatic's bedroom. If asthma is troublesome a period away from the family pet is worth trying. This will usually need to be the asthmatic rather than the pet moving out for a week or two, since even if the animal goes its allergens in hair and skin scales will remain in the house for some time.

Exercise

We saw in a previous chapter that exercise may be used as a diagnostic test for asthma, looking for the airway narrowing a few minutes after a brief bout of exertion. Asthmatics will find particular problems exercising in cold and dry atmospheres. It is important for asthmatics to stay as fit as possible as this in itself reduces the problems from a given amount of exercise. So it is better to take precautions against the exercise-induced asthma than to avoid the exercise. In most cases asthmatic schoolchildren do not need to avoid games, providing the correct treatment is used.

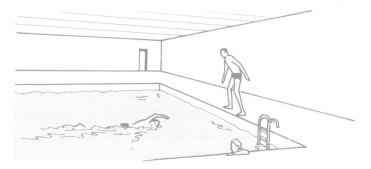

Since exercise-induced asthma seems to be connected with drying and cooling of the airways, exercising in warm, moist atmospheres is much less likely to give trouble. The best example of this is swimming in an indoor swimming pool. A few asthmatics have problems with the chemicals used in the water but otherwise this exercise is least likely to give problems. It is useful for asthmatics to warm up well at the start of exercise since in many cases with repeated bouts of exercise each successive one is less likely to give trouble.

Inhalation of a beta-agonist or sodium cromoglycate just before exercise usually abolishes the exercise-induced asthma. These treatments do not contravene the rules of sports organisations such as the International Olympic Committee and many world class athletes have achieved success despite their asthma.

Pollution

Cigarette smoke is the commonest form of air pollution that asthmatics are likely to meet, and it generally causes irritation of their sensitive airways. Surprisingly, around 15% of adult asthmatics themselves smoke. Such direct application of irritants to the airways should certainly be avoided. Exposure to other people's smoke should be avoided by keeping out of smoky atmospheres. More general air pollution, such as sulphur dioxide in factory smoke, can also cause problems. When young people with asthma are choosing a job it seems sensible for them to avoid ones where they will have to be in particularly dusty or cold atmospheres.

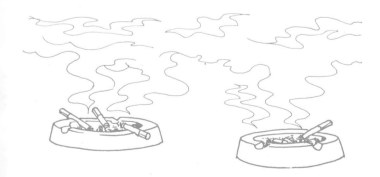

The weather

The weather can affect asthmatic airways either by changes in temperature and humidity or by changes in the number of airborne pollen grains and spores or other pollutants. In Birmingham in July 1983, after a thunderstorm and a heavy fall of rain there was a tenfold increase in the usual number of asthma admissions. This may have been due either to increases in fungal spores or to changes in pressure and humidity but it certainly shows that asthmatics may be substantially affected by the weather.

Medical treatment

Occasionally the very treatment that is being used to try to improve asthma can itself cause the airways to narrow. Fortunately this is uncommon and is usually because of rare sensitivity reactions, preservatives in the treatment, or the irritant effect of dry powder inhalations.

Some drugs will cause problems in nearly all asthmatics who take them. Beta blocker drugs are used for the treatment of high blood pressure and for heart disease. They have exactly the opposite reaction to treatments such as salbutamol and terbutaline, which widen the airways, and they can cause severe and even fatal attacks of asthma. Some of these beta blockers are designed to have most of their action on the heart rather than the airways but they can all cause trouble in asthmatics. Beta blockers may be used as eye drops in the treatment of glaucoma and even these can provoke asthma.

Some asthmatics, mainly adults, are sensitive to the aspirin group of drugs. The same problems occur with aspirin-like drugs. These are the non-steroidal anti-inflammatory drugs which are used for arthritis. Most are only available on prescription from doctors but aspirin and ibuprofen (Brufen) can be bought in a chemist without prescription. Asthmatics who are sensitive to aspirin should remember that many commercial cold cures and cough mixtures also contain it.

Sleep

The phenomenon of 'morning dipping' was described on p. 37. The problem cannot be avoided by breaking up sleep and people on shift work who sleep during the day find that the timing of the trouble changes within two or three days. The variation of the asthma throughout the day and night is best treated by improved asthma treatment throughout the 24 hours. If this fails to control the problem then it may be necessary to give some treatment aimed at covering the early hours of the morning. This will often need to be bronchodilator tablets which are taken before going to sleep and which slowly release their active constituents throughout the night.

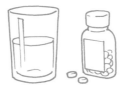

Occupation

It has long been recognised that asthma may be brought on by conditions at work, and in 1982 occupational asthma became a compensatable occupational disease in the UK. Compensation applies only to specific recognised substances and does not apply to general irritation from dust or pollution. It applies only to those who develop their asthma while in the employment and not to those who had asthma which was made worse in the job.

If factors at work are thought to be important in asthma the usual course is to make frequent recordings of peak flow rate at work and at home. Responses to factors at work may occur within minutes or be delayed until the evening or night after. A weekend away from work may not be enough to get rid of the pattern which has developed during the working week. It may be necessary to carry on the recordings during a two week holiday away from the job.

If you think that work factors may be involved in your asthma you should seek your doctor's help in investigating this since the charts of peak flow at work and at home may be quite difficult to analyse.

Food

'Food allergy' is a topic that tends to evoke strong reactions among doctors and some patients. 'Food intolerance' is usually preferred as a term to describe this as in many cases the reaction is not really an allergy involving an antibody response but is just a direct effect of some chemical component or additive in the food. The foods most commonly connected with asthmatic reactions are dairy products, nuts, alcoholic drinks, fizzy drinks and colourings such as tartrazine.

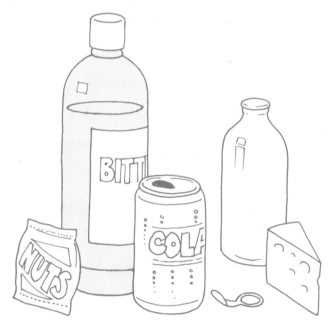

If the reactions occur within minutes they can easily be seen to be related to food but such reactions are uncommon. Later reactions are more difficult to prove. They are probably not very common, and it is only rarely that an asthmatic person needs to stick to a strict diet. Any food which is suspected should be removed from the diet for around two weeks and then introduced in small quantities. Subjective feelings about relationships to food are best backed up by peak flow recordings.

Psychological factors

It is sometimes suggested that asthmatics tend to be of a particular temperament: anxious and introverted. There is no evidence at all that this is true. What is clear is that emotional and psychological changes can affect asthma in the same way as all the other factors considered in this chapter can. Sometimes this has an obvious physical explanation. Laughter makes you take deep breaths which themselves can cause the airways to narrow. Emotions can affect how much of a feeling of shortness of breath an asthmatic has.

Changes in the airways can be induced by suggestion. If an asthmatic is told that he or she is being given an inhalation of a bronchodilator this will often result in widening of the airways even if the substance is inactive.

The changes in airway size caused by emotional and psychological factors are generally relatively small compared with the effects of allergens and other stimuli. In an acute asthma attack asthmatic patients often seem anxious but this is the result of the acute attack and not the cause of it. The anxiety is relieved by treatment of the asthma and not by sedation.

Laughter may affect asthma.

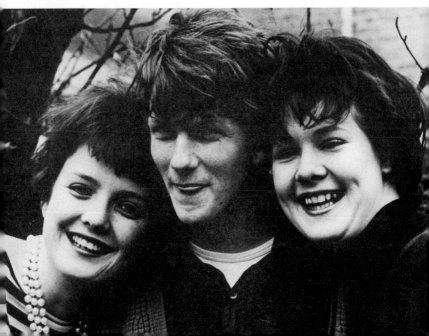

Pregnancy and menstruation

The effect of pregnancy on asthma varies from person to person. Half of the time the asthma is unaffected by the pregnancy, 30% of women are better and around 20% are worse; it may be the same in each pregnancy for some women but not for others. Fortunately there are no particular problems with asthma treatment during pregnancy and pregnant women can have the same treatment as when they are not pregnant. There may be problems if asthma is very severe and the amount of oxygen in the blood is decreased but with proper treatment there is no extra risk for the mother or the baby.

Some women find that their asthma varies with the menstrual cycle. Asthma may feel different at different times through the month even though the measurements of the amount of airway narrowing remain the same. This is perhaps because hormonal changes affect the sensation of breathlessness in the brain.

Heartburn

Some asthmatics experience problems when there is reflux of acid up into the gullet or oesophagus. This may be because of irritation around the larynx if the acid gets right to the top of the oesophagus or it may be a message sent up the nerves from the lower part of the gullet. This leak of acid up from the stomach is more likely to occur on lying down at night and may be the cause of trouble during the night in a few people. It can be treated with drugs.

7 Measurement of asthma

Asthma, as we know, is a disease that varies a lot, and objective measurements are needed to diagnose it and to monitor the effects of treatment, changing it if necessary.

The peak expiratory flow rate is the fastest rate that air can be blown out of the lungs. It can be measured on various devices. It comes near the start of blowing out when the lungs are still full of air so you just need to take a full breath in and give a short sharp blow without fully emptying the lungs.

Meter

The usual machine used for measuring peak flow rate in hospital is the Wright's peak flow meter. The reading is in litres of air per minute and is likely to be between 60 and 600. A low reading version is also available. The normal reading depends on age, height and sex. Highest readings are found at the age of 30 to 35 years and slowly decline after this.

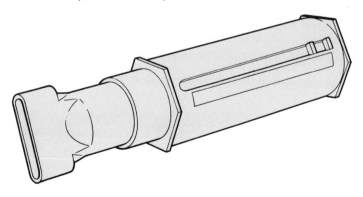

Keep a regular check

Occasional readings on a peak flow meter at the hospital or surgery are much less valuable than regular recording at home. This can be done with one of the portable peak flow meters such as the mini Wright's peak flow meter. These cost around £10 and can be obtained through hospitals, general practitioners, or the Asthma Society. They are a great benefit for most asthmatics. There may be small differences between the readings obtained on standard peak flow meters and the mini meters so that comparisons should always be made with the same instrument. Low reading varieties are available for children and those who never achieve normal flows.

To use the mini meter you must hold it horizontal with the fingers off the scale. Then take in a full breath and, with the lips tightly round the mouth piece, let out a sharp, short breath. (If you have false teeth it may be easier if you take them out before blowing.) You then read off the scale to the nearest 10 litres per minute. You return the pointer to zero and take two more readings. Asthmatics often find that the first reading is the best because the deep inspiration temporarily increases the airway narrowing and produces lower values. The best of the three results is recorded.

Uses of meters

There are many uses for peak flow recordings. They can be used to look for diurnal variation as a diagnostic test. They can be used to assess the effects of changes in treatment. Most importantly they can be used in the day to day monitoring of asthma. A regular peak flow chart recorded morning and evening before any regular treatment will give a good idea of how well the asthma is being controlled. It will give an early warning of deterioration often before other symptoms are particularly evident. This means that early action can be taken to avoid an acute attack.

Spirometry

A slightly more complex machine will look at flow rates throughout blowing out. The commonest sort of machine is a dry bellows into which you must breathe, pushing all the air out until the lungs are empty. Two main measurements are taken. One is the volume of air blown out in the first second (FEV1 = forced expiratory volume in one second) and the other is the total volume of air blown out (FVC = forced vital capacity). Normally about three quarters of the total volume can be blown out in the first second but in asthma where the airways are narrowed this ratio (FEV1/FVC) is reduced.

Other lung function tests

Sometimes other lung function tests are useful. Testing for over-responsiveness has already been mentioned (p. 38). The lungs get larger as asthma gets worse, and the total volume of air in the lungs, even that which cannot be blown out, can be measured by breathing air containing a little helium or by making measurements inside a closed box, the body plethysmograph. Some of these extra tests may be useful in picking up some diagnostic problems in suspected asthma such as the obstruction in a large airway.

Peak flow cards

Charts are available for monitoring asthma at home. The simple way is just to write down each day, or plot on a graph, the peak flow results. It is helpful also to have records of symptoms and of inhaler use. Some charts are quite complicated and it needs a lot of time and effort to complete them regularly. Since most of my patients are not so obsessional I prefer a simpler chart where peak flow can be recorded together with a space for comments. The patient is asked to write in the comment column anything relevant such as increased inhaler use, cough or night-time waking.

Patterns of peak flow at home

The recording of peak flow at home shows various different patterns some of which are illustrated in the case histories that follow. The peak flow records are shown in a graph.

Case history — Sarah

Sarah is now 21 and has had asthma for 15 years. Various factors bring on attack but particularly any respiratory tract infections. She has not had any infections recently but her asthma has been difficult to control. She is taking high doses of inhaled salbutamol, and inhaled steroids as well as theophylline tablets.

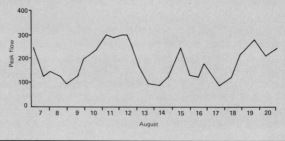

Comment

Sarah has a chaotic looking peak flow chart with no real pattern to it, it just swings up and down violently. This is sometimes known as brittle asthma and is often quite difficult to get under good control.

Case history — Harry

Harry has had asthma since he was 6 years old, 60 years ago. He has had increasing problems with his breathing and his inhalers seem to be less useful than they were.

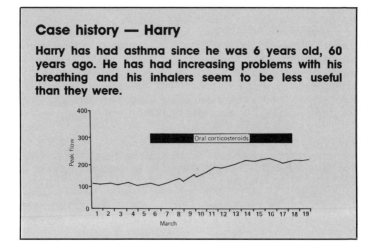

Comment

The peak flow chart shows consistently low values with little daily or day to day variation. This situation may improve with a trial of a short course of oral corticosteroids.

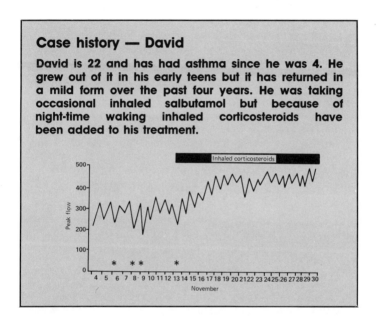

Case history — David

David is 22 and has had asthma since he was 4. He grew out of it in his early teens but it has returned in a mild form over the past four years. He was taking occasional inhaled salbutamol but because of night-time waking inhaled corticosteroids have been added to his treatment.

Comment

The peak flow chart shows a typical asthmatic variation and the stars on the chart show nights when David was woken by his asthma. The addition of inhaled corticosteroids has produced some improvement over two weeks. There is still daily variation in peak flow but because it is happening at a higher level it is not resulting in waking at night. Although the symptoms are better, the continued variation throughout the day suggests that David's airways are still over-responsive and if this does not settle he may have to take larger doses of the inhaled steroid or additional drugs. This is obvious from the peak flow chart but might have been missed on the symptoms alone.

Case history — Vicky

Vicky has had asthma for 30 years and she is now 35. She normally takes inhaled salbutamol and sodium cromoglycate and has few problems. She has had seven previous admissions to hospital and now keeps a supply of oral corticosteroids and antibiotics at home. Recently she developed a sore throat which went on to give her a cough and to make her wheezy. Her peak flow rate dropped from its usual levels of around 400 litres per minute to 250 litres per minute and she started her oral corticosteroids and her antibiotics. The peak flow started to rise within 24 hours and in five days it was back up to its usual levels. Vicky made an appointment to see her general practitioner when she started taking the steroids but when she saw him two days later the asthma was improving.

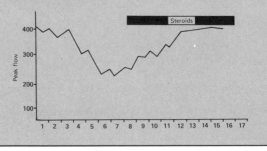

Comment

Vicky has learnt from her previous attacks that they are usually preceded by some days of deterioration. She has worked out a plan of action with her doctor based on her symptoms and her peak flow results. When these reached her threshold of 250 litres per minute she started her steroids, the peak flow rose, and she avoided another admission to hospital.

8 Coping with asthma

Most patients who have asthma will need some drug treatment at least some of the time. There will be a few patients who can avoid drug treatment by staying away from the triggers which bring on their asthma but these fortunate individuals are definitely in the minority. Most asthma drug treatments are remarkably safe but should still only be taken if necessary. It is important to understand the reasons for the regimen of treatment that your doctor has chosen for you.

It is possible just to follow a list of treatments without understanding the reasons behind it just as you would follow a recipe. The problem is that the dish only varies if the recipe is not followed while asthma varies of its own accord and the ingredients of the recipe may have to be changed to deal with its variation.

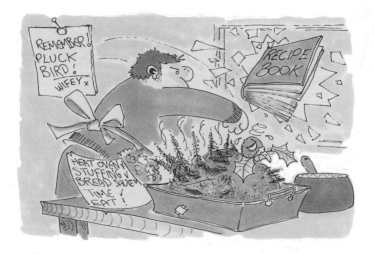

This does not mean that asthma can only be coped with successfully by those with a degree in pharmacology. It just requires a broad understanding of the different treatment groups, to know which one to adjust in different circumstances, and when to seek further help. The various groups of asthma treatments will be covered in the following chapters.

Avoiding asthma without drugs

On p. 42 the numerous factors that may provoke asthma were discussed and we saw that most asthmatics have irritable airways that respond to a wide variety of different stimuli. Some asthmatic patients have just one trigger which sets off their asthma or at least one factor to which they are most sensitive. If this is an allergen such as cat fur or a certain food or drink then it can be avoided without too much difficulty by most people. When it is an unusual allergen but contact with it occurs as part of your job the situation is more difficult. Extra precautions at work or even a change of job may be necessary (occupational asthma is described on p. 49).

Nevertheless, the two most common triggers of asthma in the UK are house dust mites and grass pollen. Contact can be reduced by sensible precautions but complete avoidance is not practical. The sensible precautions may even have their own advantages: asthma can provide an excellent excuse to avoid housework and mowing the lawn. We know that complete removal from all exposure to house dust mites is effective but it is difficult to prove that this sort of sensible, modest reduction in contact with known allergens is really beneficial. However, it seems likely to go some way towards reducing the inflammation (p. 18) in the airways and, therefore, reducing the general responsiveness to other triggers.

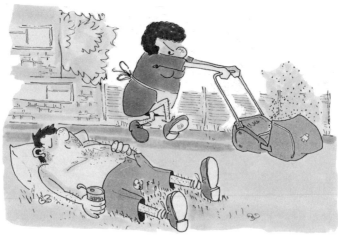

Exercise

It is important to remember that this sort of approach of avoiding known provoking factors does not apply to exercise-induced asthma. Exercise does not increase general twitchiness of the airways in the same way as allergic responses. Although exercise-induced asthma should be avoided as much as possible by a warm up before exercise and by suitable drug treatment, exercise itself is to be encouraged. Fit people do not get out of breath so quickly whether they are asthmatic or not.

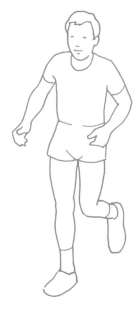

Some of the other non-drug treatments that have been used for asthma are described on p. 80. They may be helpful for some people but they are not usually enough to control asthma satisfactorily on their own, without drug treatment.

Determining triggers

When you give an account of your asthma to your doctor you should try to describe any specific situations in which it has been provoked. Then you can both try to discover the relevant provoking factors. The importance of these triggers may be then backed up by skin prick tests or blood tests for specific antibodies (p. 41).

General approach to drug treatment

The following chapters will describe the various drugs available for the treatment of asthma. In general, drugs fall into two categories. The first of these is the bronchodilator group of drugs. These are used to widen airways that are already narrowed in an attack of asthma. You can also take them before contact with some asthma triggers and they will often stop the asthma being provoked. The second group of drugs can prevent asthma if they are taken before contact with a trigger but are of no use if they are given to try to reverse narrowing of the airways when it has already happened. The most widely used drugs in this group are sodium cromoglycate and inhaled corticosteroids.

Which drugs?

There is a general feeling among most doctors interested in asthma that it is not enough simply to keep the airways open by responding to symptoms with bronchodilators or even to use bronchodilators alone to prevent narrowing of the airways. This treatment does not deal with the inflammation in the walls of the airways which keeps up their responsiveness. There has therefore, been a widespread move towards the use of the second group of drugs described above in any patients who have frequent symptoms. There is some limited evidence to support this approach and it certainly seems to be logical. Doctors vary in how severe they think the asthma should be before it is right to move on from bronchodilators alone to other continuous treatment.

Know your treatment

The first thing to know about the treatment you use for your asthma is whether it can be varied to cope with changes in your symptoms. If a mild attack of wheeziness comes on you can generally put a stop to it with a couple of puffs of bronchodilator, but an extra puff or two of inhaled corticosteroid (such as Becotide, Pulmicort) or sodium cromoglycate (such as Intal) will be useless.

Mild asthmatics may not need regular treatment at all and will be able to manage with a supply of bronchodilator to use when symptoms arise or before known triggers such as exercise. Most other asthmatics will have regular treatment, which they must remember to take every day if their asthma is giving no trouble, and extra treatment which they take when their asthma gets worse. The extra treatment may also be part of their regular treatment.

Every asthmatic must know:

- **In general terms what each of the treatments does;**
- **How to adjust the treatment if asthma gets worse;**
- **How to avoid asthma by treatment or other means;**
- **What to do if usual treatment fails to work;**
- **How to get extra help quickly;**
- **When to seek the extra help.**

Work out a plan

Asthma is unpredictable. The time to learn what to do if an acute attack comes on is before it happens, not when lying in hospital recovering from a severe attack, which could have been prevented with earlier action. Remember that most acute asthma attacks are preceded by plenty of warnings as the asthma slowly gets worse. The time for action is during this early deterioration; it is much easier and safer to control the asthma at this point than to wait for the acute severe attack and try to reverse it. A few asthmatic patients have very sudden attacks which are not preceded by such a slow worsening. These attacks are more difficult to deal with but it is even more important to work out beforehand a plan of action to cope with them than for the usual asthmatic attack after slow worsening.

9 Types of drugs for asthma

A bronchodilator is a drug which increases the diameter of the airways over a short period, thus reducing the resistance to the passage of air in and out while you breathe. It acts partly by relaxing the smooth muscle in the wall of the airways; but it also cuts down release of harmful mediators and has an effect on the inflammation in the airway wall.

> **Bronchodilators are given for two main reasons, either to reverse airway narrowing which has already occurred or to prevent the effect of some sort of asthma trigger.**

Bronchodilators

There are three main groups of bronchodilators available. The first group is the beta-adrenergic drugs which act in the same sort of way as the body's natural hormone, adrenaline. Alterations in their chemical structure have restricted the action to the lungs rather than the more general stimulating actions of adrenaline. These are the most widely used bronchodilator drugs.

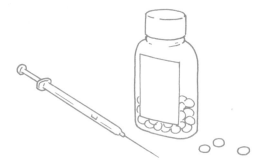

Anticholinergics

The second group is the anticholinergic drugs. These act by blocking the signal to constrict the airways that comes from the main nerve supply to the lung running in the vagus nerve.

Xanthine derivatives

The third group of bronchodilators are the xanthine derivatives. These are drugs with similar properties to caffeine, the active ingredient in coffee. Unlike the other groups they are not taken by inhalation but in tablets or by injection.

Beta-adrenergic bronchodilators

Beta-adrenergic bronchodilators are the commonest form of bronchodilators used in asthma and, indeed, the commonest of all the groups of asthma drugs. The drugs which are most often prescribed in this group are salbutamol, terbutaline, and fenoterol. Adrenaline itself has been used for many years in the treatment of asthma, usually as an injection during an acute attack. Adrenaline has much more effect in stimulating the heart than the newer drugs, which are safer because they have their major effects on the lungs rather than the heart. However, even drugs such as salbutamol and terbutaline can produce a speeding up of the heart in some people.

Instruction is needed in the use of aerosol inhalers.

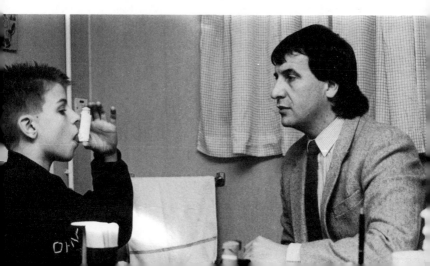

How to take them

The beta-adrenergic drugs can be taken by inhalation, nebuliser, tablets or injection. Injections are used occasionally for severe attacks of asthma. A few patients have such persistent troublesome asthma that they have been treated at home with a slow continuous trickle of drug from a battery-driven pump under the skin.

There is a very small minority of patients who have such severe attacks of asthma with no warning that they are at great risk from the sudden swings in their asthma. These patients can be given a pre-loaded syringe to keep always with them and can be taught to inject the drug under the skin or into the muscle of the leg in an emergency.

The use of injected drugs is usually a desperate measure and inhaled and oral treatments are much more commonly used. In general inhaling the treatment directly into the lungs is preferable. This has the advantages that the dose can be kept low and side effects avoided because the drug goes straight to the site where it has to act rather than being distributed throughout the different tissues in the body. A disadvantage of tablets is that they are much slower to act. An inhaler will start to improve asthma within five minutes while a tablet will not start to work for 30 to 60 minutes.

Tablets may be useful for night-time asthma since they can have a longer action than the currently available inhaled bronchodilators. It is sometimes useful to take a slow-acting drug before going to bed so that the effect is maintained throughout the night.

Inhalers

There are three main ways of inhaling bronchodilator drugs, metered dose inhalers, dry powder systems, and nebulisers. The commonest device used to administer an inhaled drug is a *metered dose inhaler*. These inhalers produce a fine mist which can be inhaled. This must be done carefully (see box). Even after instruction some patients find it very difficult to inhale adequately from the metered dose inhalers and most doctors like to check on inhaler technique periodically.

Common problems with metered dose inhalers are not shaking the canister properly to disperse the drug, activating the inhaler after breathing in and stopping breathing in when the cold jet reaches the back of the mouth. Even if your inhalation technique is perfect, a lot of the fast jet from the

The technique of using a metered dose inhaler:

- **Shake the canister;**
- **Take off the protective cap;**
- **Hold the inhaler between the lips;**
- **Breathe out;**
- **Take a long slow breath in;**
- **Actuate the inhaler near the start of this deep breathing in;**
- **Continue to breathe in until the lungs are full;**
- **Hold the breath and count slowly to 10;**
- **Breathe out and wait one minute before a second inhalation.**

inhaler hits the back of the mouth and this is then swallowed. Only around one tenth of the output of the inhaler actually gets down in to the lungs where it has its effect.

If you have problems

Some patients with arthritic hands cannot fire the inhalers and can be helped by devices which just need to be squeezed. Several other methods are available if you have problems with a metered dose inhaler:

An extension tube on the inhaler These vary from short tubes to large plastic globes which get over nearly all the problems of coordination between hands and breathing. The inhaler is actuated into the globe and the breath can then be taken through the valve on the mouthpiece. This technique also helps to stop most of the inhaler going in the mouth instead of the lungs, and produces smaller particles in the mist which get in to the lungs more efficiently.

Breath triggered inhalers To try to help people get the coordination needed to use an inhaler some of these are made to act automatically when they are sucked through. Some patients find them useful but they can make you breathe in too fast and the sudden automatic firing of the inhaler can stop you breathing in.

A dry powder

The advantage of this is that the airflow which sends the drug into the lungs is produced by the patient's own breathing in, rather than a pressurised inhaler. It requires a fast sucking breath through the device and then a breath-hold for 10 seconds. One disadvantage of these devices was that they used to have to be loaded up for each dose and this made them a little less convenient than the spray form of inhaler. The ingenious manufacturers have now come up with new devices which contain multiple doses and get over this problem.

Nebulisers

Asthmatic patients who are admitted to hospital because of their asthma are usually treated with a nebuliser. There are two sorts of nebuliser: an ultrasonic variety and the commoner form of jet nebuliser which is powered by a stream of air. The cloud of nebulised drug is taken through a facemask or a mouthpiece. The advantage of the nebuliser is that the treatment is taken in during normal breathing and this avoids all the coordination problems of the other devices. Two disadvantages are that nebulisers are expensive and require a power supply. They are unnecessary for most asthmatics and they do have a potential danger in that asthmatic people may stay at home during an acute attack using a nebuliser when they really need other treatment or hospital care. Most doctors are therefore, reluctant to sanction the use of nebulisers at home

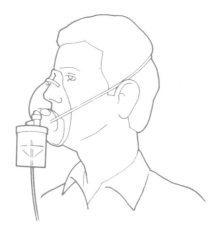

> **Home nebulisers may be used for:**
>
> - **Patients who are unable to cope with any other inhaler (unusual with spacer devices now available);**
> - **Young children (dry powder inhalers can be used from about 4 years of age and spacer devices before that);**
> - **Patients who need high doses of bronchodilator (the nebuliser dose is usually much higher than the other inhaler doses);**
> - **Patients who have acute attacks of asthma. Great care must be taken in using nebulisers in these circumstances. Acute attacks of asthma can be fatal and the nebuliser must be part of a carefully prepared plan of action. It most not delay the use of other appropriate measures.**

without good reasons and unless they are confident that their patient has a good understanding of the management of his or her asthma.

Anticholinergic bronchodilators

Anticholinergic drugs have been used in asthma for many years. They formed the active ingredient of asthma cigarettes which were once popular. The most widely available treatment in this group is ipratropium bromide (Atrovent) which can be taken by inhaler or by nebuliser. These bronchodilators block the contraction of smooth muscle which occurs through signals in the vagus nerve.

In most asthmatic people anticholinergic drugs are not as effective as the beta-adrenergic group described above. There are, however, some circumstances in which they can be useful: such as for very young children (under 18 months) and for older people. Anticholinergic drugs take effect more slowly than the adrenergic drugs, taking 30 to 60 minutes to achieve the maximum effect, but the effect lasts rather longer.

69

Xanthine derivatives

Caffeine, the active ingredient of coffee, is a xanthine derivative and is a mild bronchodilator. Theophylline and its soluble salt, aminophylline, are more often used for treatment. They are not effective when inhaled and are available in three forms — as tablets, injections, and suppositories. Suppositories are absorbed at an unreliable rate which means that the effect is unpredictable. Injections are used for acute severe asthma and tablets are used for bronchodilatation for people with chronic asthma.

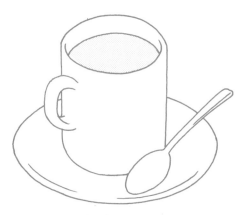

Bronchodilators act by widening the airways in the lungs. There are three groups of bronchodilators:

- **adrenergic drugs**
- **anticholinergics**
- **the xanthine group.**

The first two groups are taken by inhaling and the dose may be regular or adjusted to deal with any symptoms that arise. Xanthines are given as tablets; the dose must be carefully controlled and not adjusted to the symptoms.

Treatment needs monitoring

The way xanthines produce widening of the airways is uncertain. The dose given needs to be carefully controlled because when the level in the blood is above the range where the effect occurs, side effects such as sickness can occur. The dose needed to produce the effect is unpredictable in any one person and is best guided by measurement of the level of theophylline in the blood. Theophylline treatment needs to be taken continuously at the dose which has been established by the blood tests. It is important to remember that it should not be adjusted in line with symptoms in the same way as inhaled bronchodilators.

Many drugs as well as other illnesses and smoking can alter the level of theophylline in the blood and so care must be taken when other treatments are combined with theophyllines.

Most tablets are designed to slowly release the theophylline which they contain. This allows them to have a prolonged effect and makes them particularly useful for controlling night-time asthma.

10 Long-term treatment for asthma

We have seen earlier that the recognition by doctors of the importance of persistent inflammation in the walls of the airways in asthma has led them to change their approach to the treatment. Rather than be satisfied with a widening of the airways with bronchodilators there is a widespread feeling that it may be more important to try to suppress the inflammation. Several drugs are available for this purpose.

Sodium cromoglycate

It has long been thought that sodium cromoglycate (Intal) works by reducing the body's allergic reactions, though recently it has been suggested that it may have an effect on the nerve endings which cause reflex narrowing of the airways.

One great advantage of sodium cromoglycate is that it is virtually free of side effects apart from occasional irritation of the throat from the dry powder version. It is available as a dry powder, as an inhaler or as a nebuliser solution.

Helps children and young adults

Sodium cromoglycate is most likely to be effective in children and young adults whose symptoms are known to be partly due to a specific allergy. It is less likely to help adults. You can use it specifically to avoid exercise induced asthma by taking it 15 minutes before exercise but in general it must be taken continuously to be of use. In the past it was usually taken as dry powder from a spinhaler four times a day but a simpler inhaled version is now available and is used by the method shown on p. 67. You need to take sodium cromoglycate continuously for six weeks before deciding whether it is effective.

Takes time to work

When drugs in this category do work they improve the symptoms of asthma and cut down the need for bronchodilator treatment. Once control has been established the dose of sodium cromoglycate can be maintained or gradually reduced to find a plateau below which mild symptoms break through. Preventive medicines such as sodium cromoglycate should be taken for six to 12 months before you try to stop them, as it is hoped that prolonged reduction in the airway inflammation will have long term beneficial effects.

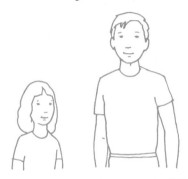

Nedocromil sodium

A more recent product is nedocromil sodium (Tilade). This has similar properties to sodium cromoglycate but may have more of an attack on the inflammation in the airway wall than on the allergic component. It is also taken by inhaling two or four times a day. Some patients find that nedocromil has a bitter taste. Just like sodium cromoglycate it is used as continuous long term treatment in addition to bronchodilators as necessary.

Corticosteroids

The mention of steroid treatment worries most patients. Most will have heard of the harmful effects of long term treatment. However, continuous treatment with corticosteroid tablets for asthma is unusual. It is resorted to only when most other safer treatments have failed.

This worry about steroids often extends unnecessarily to two other kinds of drug which are very important in the modern treatment of asthma. These are inhaled steroids and short courses of steroid tablets.

Inhaled corticosteroids

Inhaled corticosteroids have very few side effects. This is because they are applied directly to the lining of the airways and very little of the drug gets into the rest of the body. They can be taken in the same way as beta-adrenergic bronchodilators by using a metered dose inhaler with or without a spacing device or a dry powder system.

Inhaled steroids are of little or no use in acute severe attacks of asthma and are used for long term preventive treatment in the same way as sodium cromoglycate. The effect of an inhaled steroid may take some weeks to become noticeable once treatment has started. Its use can be limited to twice a day in most patients. This helps to distinguish it from the bronchodilator which is usually used when it is needed. A typical patient can have a steroid inhaler by the bedside to use on getting up and going to bed and a bronchodilator to carry around all day and use as it is needed. An episode of acute asthma should be treated with the bronchodilator.

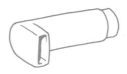

Side effects of inhaled corticosteroids

The worrying side effects of oral steroids are not seen at all with inhaled steroids. If the dose is very large then it is possible to show on blood tests that enough of the drug is getting into the general system to be detectable but not to cause any problems. It is possible that very high doses in children might affect growth, but this does not occur at usual doses and is less of a problem than the effects of uncontrolled asthma.

The adverse effects of the inhaled steroids are around the mouth. The voice may be a little husky; an infection of the mouth and throat with a fungus (candidiasis or thrush) affects less than one in 20 patients. Thrush is less common if the dose is kept down to two rather than four times a day. Rarely, there is an effect on the vocal cords which causes a weak voice. These local effects are caused by the steroid in the mouth, which is of no use in treating the asthma. They can be lessened by increasing the amount entering the lungs and reducing that lost in the mouth. This can be achieved with a spacing device (p. 67). When thrush has appeared in the mouth a short course of antifungal lozenges or pastilles may be necessary.

Oral corticosteroids

Although continuously taking corticosteroids causes all sorts of skin, bone, and weight problems, short courses for two to three weeks have very few side effects. They are often used when asthma has been gradually getting worse. They are also given for acute, severe asthma, sometimes by injection into a vein. They take six hours or more to begin to achieve their effect.

Most studies of deaths and disasters from asthma have identified *a reluctance* on the part of the doctor and the patients to use oral corticosteroids as a very important factor.

Steroids are an essential part of the treatment of asthma and many patients keep an emergency supply at home. They can start these without delay and then be assessed to see if further action is needed. In these cases careful plans of action must be set up so that the patients are confident in the use of their steroids. Home peak flow recording is usually very helpful.

The dose of corticosteroids used for a short course varies. Most doctors give 20 to 40 mg daily as a single, morning dose. This is given for 10 to 21 days and then stopped. Sometimes the dose may be tailed off over five or six days.

When steroids are used for longer periods your doctor will usually try to minimise the effects by reducing the dose to one day in two, taken in the morning, and giving inhaled steroids to help keep the oral dose as low as possible.

Ketotifen

Ketotifen is taken in tablet form as regular drug treatment. It is an antihistamine which also has some antiallergic properties. It may be helpful for some patients, but the disadvantage is that the antihistamine may cause drowsiness.

Choosing the drug for prevention

There is little evidence that combining the preventive medicines just described has any great benefit. Generally a single drug will be chosen. For children whose allergic elements are troublesome, sodium cromoglycate is the best first choice. For older patients the first choice lies between inhaled cortico-steroids and nedocromil sodium for mild disease, with inhaled steroids for moderate problems.

Take them regularly

The important aspect of these treatments is that they only work if they are taken regularly, supplemented by bronchodilators as necessary. The commonest reasons for failure of such treatment are that the inhalation technique is poor or that the asthmatic doesn't remember to take the drug regularly.

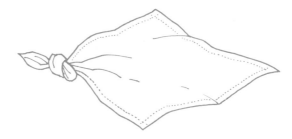

Is it working?

The responses need to be measured in some way, preferably by daily readings of peak flow rate which can be measured at home. The patient and doctor must then decide on the level at which the patient must seek further help (such as oral steroid treatment) because routine treatment is failing. Results of home peak flow recording have shown that inhaled steroids work well controlling asthma in most patients.

11 Avoiding allergens, and desensitisation

Apart from drug treatment, there are two potential ways to deal with the allergic problems of asthma. We have already seen that the commonest inhaled allergens such as grass pollens and the house dust mite are very common and consequently difficult to avoid. Nevertheless, efforts should certainly be made to reduce contact with these allergens. A few patients have specific problems with one or two less common antigens and they may be able to avoid them.

Asthmatic patients should also try not to develop sensitivities to new allergens that may be breathed in. This means that they should avoid most pets even if initial skin tests have suggested that they are not allergic. A negative skin test may simply show that there has not been much contact in the past. The skin tests may become positive and symptoms of asthma develop with the prolonged close contact which is certain to occur with a pet cat or dog in the house.

Case history — Mark

Eight year old Mark has had asthma for five years. A cat had been the family pet until 18 months previously when the cat had died. Mark was very anxious to have another pet although his symptoms had improved somewhat since the cat's death. He was not satisfied with the goldfish which his mother had initially bought. His mother persuaded her doctor to arrange a set of skin prick tests. Mark showed positive responses to house dust mite, grass pollen, some early tree pollens, and cat and dog fur, but no response to rabbits or other small furry animals. On the basis of this they bought two rabbits. Within two months Mark's asthma was beginning to get worse and he began to notice a connection between attacks of asthma and handling

the rabbits or cleaning their cages. Repeat skin
tests now showed similar results to those previously,
with the addition of a moderately strong reaction to
rabbit. Removal of the rabbits again produced a
slow improvement in his asthma.

Comment

This is a fairly typical story. The negative response on the first set
of skin tests is no guarantee that responses will not subsequently
occur and, predictably, symptoms gradually recurred with a
new animal. Asthmatics like Mark should try to avoid lengthy
contact with any furry animals.

Occupational problems

Occupational asthma is another condition which may be much
improved by avoiding one particular substance. Continued
contact at work may increase the asthmatic patient's reaction
to all sorts of other conditions not just the work. Thus it is
important to try to detect any work related asthma problems.

Case history — Edward

Now aged 35, Edward had had mild asthma as a
child but this had all resolved in his teenage years
and he had been free of symptoms for 20 years
before he took up his job in a paint factory. Over
the first six months of his job he began to get a
return of his asthma symptoms. This affected him
during the day at work and he also began to notice
shortness of breath and wheezing in smoky atmospheres and with exercise. After a thorough investi-
gation of his asthma he was moved to another job
in the same firm. His asthma at work went away
over two to three weeks and his troubles with dust,
smoke, and exercise disappeared over the next
month.

Comment

Edward already had an underlying tendency to have asthma. Something at work, probably chemicals called di-isocyanates, sparked this off again. Not only did he have trouble at work but his airways became generally irritable again so that they responded to all sorts of other stimuli. When he was removed from the sensitising substance at work all the other problems improved. Sometimes it may take much longer than this for the asthma to settle down after removal from contact.

Hyposensitisation and immunotherapy

For the past 80 years doctors have been trying to change the allergic responses of asthmatic patients. The most popular approach has been hyposensitisation or desensitisation. Small amounts of the troublesome substance are given to try to get the body's immune system to develop a tolerance to that substance and so stop the asthmatic response. The same approach has been widely used for hay fever with a series of injections in the early spring just before the pollen season.

In asthma, hyposensitisation has most often been tried for sensitivities to grass pollen and to house dust mite. Attempts have also been made to treat it with a whole mixture of substances based on the results of skin tests. There is no evidence that this approach of multiple hyposensitisation is of any benefit at all. There is some controversy about hyposensitisation to one substance. Some studies show that there may be some benefit, but only in certain patients and greater benefit can usually be achieved by fairly simple inhaler treatment.

Questionable value

A course of treatment consists of regular injections, slowly increasing the amount injected. Local swelling or more serious general reactions occur quite often and several deaths have occurred as a result of hyposensitisation treatment. Most deaths have resulted from some mistake in the dilution of the injection or inadequate supervision of the patient after the injection. Most doctors are therefore very cautious about hyposensitisation and will only carry out the treatment where there is adequate experience and supervision, and facilities for resuscitation. This worry and the disappointing results severely limit the value of hyposensitisation in the opinion of many doctors.

12 Alternative treatments

The previous chapter described some attempts to deal with the allergic responses of asthma without drugs. Many other treatments for asthma have been tried, with variable success. Most doctors have some problem in assessing the value of these treatments. Doctors usually prescribe treatments which have been evaluated by what are called 'double blind controlled trials'. This means that neither the doctor nor the patient knows whether the treatment they are receiving is the new one being evaluated or not. It will be compared with another treatment known to be effective or with an inactive treatment; in drug trials this would be a dummy tablet or placebo. All commonly used asthma drugs have shown their value in this sort of research study, and many asthma patients have helped by agreeing to be volunteers in these research studies.

In asthma it is particularly important to perform these studies because we know that the state of a patient's asthma can be affected by suggestion. If we give an inactive inhaler and tell the patient it is going to improve their asthma then it will often have some beneficial or 'placebo' effect. It is, therefore, difficult to know what to make of reports that a new treatment is successful unless it has been properly assessed. New drugs can easily be tested in this way but it is not nearly so easy to use these methods for some of the non-drug treatments; a patient having hypnotherapy or doing yoga will know which treatment group he or she is in. Controlled trials of acupuncture have been possible by using different sites or not vibrating the needles.

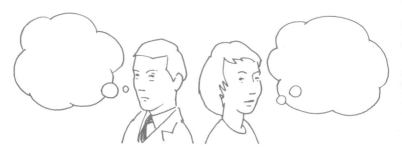

This lack of controlled evidence means that most doctors would bring in a 'not proven' verdict on many of the non-drug treatments at present. Certainly there is little to suggest that any of them have a very profound effect on asthma or can compare with conventional drug treatment. They may have a mild effect and whether this is real or through the patient's own belief in the treatment does not really matter as long as it does not delay the start of effective and necessary drug treatment if asthma becomes more severe.

Hypnosis

When asthmatic patients become anxious they tend to take bigger breaths and this can make their asthma worse. The ability to relax in these circumstances may well be beneficial for asthma, and hypnotherapy may help in this. Some studies suggest that hypnotherapy can be helpful for some patients.

Yoga

One large study from India has shown a small benefit from traditional yoga techniques. It may also help by teaching the ability to relax in stressful situations such as asthma.

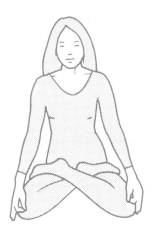

Acupuncture

There are various asthma and lung points which have been used in Chinese acupuncture for many years in the treatment of asthma, particularly Tiantu on the front of the neck, Dingchuan at the side of the neck, and Lieque on the arm. Some studies have suggested that acupuncture may alter the effect of some drugs or change how breathless a patient feels with a certain degree of asthma.

Homoeopathy

Homoeopathy entails giving minute amounts of substances which in larger amounts would produce the same symptoms as the condition being treated. These substances are diluted so much that it is difficult to believe that there are enough molecules left to have any possible effect. Homoeopathic remedies could easily be evaluated in the controlled trials discussed above but there is no such scientific evidence that they are effective in asthma. On the other hand they are unlikely to be harmful unless they are used at the expense of conventional, effective treatment.

Ionisers

Small machines that produce negative ions from the air are widely advertised for the treatment of asthma. There is no good evidence that they help.

Breathing exercises

Breathing exercises may help in teaching relaxation, and in one controlled study breathing exercises and hypnosis produced the same effects.

Herbal remedies

Many substances are used in the various herbal 'cures' for the treatment of asthma. Some of them are effective because they contain the same substances as conventional asthma drugs. A few preparations have even been found to contain large doses of corticosteroids! Naturally these are effective but have all the side effects mentioned on p. 75.

Exercise

Exercise is one of the factors that may bring on asthma, but unlike other triggers it should not be avoided. When exercise induces asthma it does not lead to increased problems with other factors. In fact, a second exercise up to two hours after the first will often fail to provoke asthma. This protection can be used by athletes with a brief warm up before full exercise. Exercise-induced asthma can also be prevented by use of drugs such as bronchodilators, or sodium cromoglycate beforehand. It is important that asthmatic patients should exercise, try to stay fit, and not become overweight.

13 Acute asthma

There are still too many deaths from asthma every year in most countries and, of course, these deaths follow acute attacks of asthma. These severe attacks may occur 'out of the blue' but more often they are preceded by periods of poor asthma control. Although most acute attacks of asthma are followed by satisfactory recovery, they are best avoided. Many of them could be avoided by proper changes in treatment during the period of deterioration before the acute attack.

Detecting deterioration

The phase of worsening asthma is more likely to be reliably detected if the state of the asthma is being monitored with home recordings of the peak flow rate (p. 54). Suitable changes in treatment at this time, with a course of steroids or an adjustment of inhaled drug, are usually very effective, but treatment is likely to be much more difficult and prolonged if the asthma slips further towards a severe attack.

> **The first important message about acute asthma is to avoid it by suitable routine treatment and monitoring so that the early signs of an acute attack are noted and treatment is changed at this stage.**

Know what to do

This prevention of attacks is not always possible and the second important aspect of acute asthma is to know exactly what to do if an acute attack does come on. This should be worked out with the doctor well beforehand, even if you have never had a severe attack. Acute asthma is a very frightening condition and many asthmatics will testify that they do not always think as logically in an acute attack as when they are well. Therefore they need to have their plans well formulated and to make sure that those around them also know what needs to be done when the attack develops. Most asthmatic patients will never have severe attacks and only a small minority need hospital admission so some of these points may sound over-dramatic. However, they are well worth sorting out and if you never have to use them so much the better.

Work out your plan for coping with an acute attack well beforehand!

The plan of action for an acute attack will need to be worked out for each individual patient but there are some general rules. Always deal with the situation early rather than waiting for the asthma to worsen and then dealing with it. Early increases in treatment will usually mean less treatment in the end.

Err on the side of safety. It is better to take one extra course of steroids a year than too few and have a prolonged stay in hospital. Always make sure you have enough of the medicines. It is very important always to keep a good supply of medicines and not run out of bronchodilators at any time, but the middle of an acute attack is certainly not the best time. Make sure of this by always keeping a spare inhaler and getting a new one from the doctor each time a new inhaler is started, not when it is running out. Many patients keep their own steroid drugs at home so they can start to take them when their symptoms or peak flows reach a certain point.

Look out for failing treatment. In acute asthma broncho-dilators may fail either by not producing relief or by their effect not lasting as long as usual. If either of these occurs then alternative treatment is needed.

Know whom to contact. Always know how to contact your general practitioner. Some hospitals have schemes through which certain asthma patients can arrange their own admission when necessary. Details of these plans will be discussed at your hospital. Remember that you can always go straight to a casualty department at any time with no appointment (make sure you know where your nearest casualty department is and whether it is open throughout 24 hours).

Home or hospital

When asthmatic patients are seen at home with acute asthma their general practitioner will decide whether treatment should be at home or in hospital. If treatment is to be at home it will often consist of a course of oral steroids, nebuliser treatment and, perhaps, an injection at the start. It is important to ensure that any initial improvement is sustained, otherwise admission to hospital may still be necessary.

In hospital various aspects of treatment may be applied:

Drug treatments

Bronchodilator treatment will usually be given by nebuliser. Injections may be given at first. These may be bronchodilators such as salbutamol or aminophylline or corticosteroid. If more than one injection is likely a needle will usually be left in a vein to allow this. It can also be used to give some extra fluid since many patients with acute asthma get rather short of fluid because they lose water from the lungs and are too short of breath to drink enough.

Oxygen

Oxygen will often be given through a mask or two flexible tubes in the nose. The need for oxygen will often be judged by blood samples taken from an artery at the wrist or the elbow.

Ventilation

For a very severe attack of asthma it may occasionally be necessary to take over the patient's breathing with a ventilator. This usually happens when the asthma is so severe that the breathing muscles begin to get over tired. The machine is connected to a tube which is placed in the windpipe or trachea through the mouth or the nose. At first the patient will be sedated and the muscles paralysed so that the patient is unaware of the machine and the tube. As recovery occurs the patient will be woken up and may breathe with the tube in place for a short time before it is removed. Such treatment is only necessary in a few very severe cases and the great majority of these patients recover from their severe attacks even if they have been bad enough to need ventilation for several days.

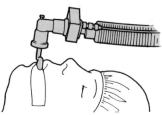

Monitoring progress

While in hospital the patient's progress will be monitored with peak flow measurements, pulse, blood pressure and the like. Few people like staying in hospital but it is important not to be in too much of a hurry to be discharged after an acute attack of asthma. The week or so after the attack is a rather vulnerable time before things really settle down again. If treatment is stopped too quickly it may just lead to another, longer admission.

Taking stock

An acute attack whether it is treated at home or in hospital should always be regarded as a time to review the usual asthma treatment, to work out why the attack occurred and how such problems might be avoided in the future. It might be a time to change the routine treatment, to learn how to deal with the early signs of deterioration, to start monitoring peak flow rate at home, or to adjust the acute crisis plan.

14 Childhood asthma

There has been a tendency for asthma to be underdiagnosed in children; often it has been labelled as bronchitis or wheezy bronchitis. This has sometimes been done to try to avoid anxiety among parents but it seems that when the actual term asthma is avoided the treatment given is often inadequate or unsuitable. Parents are more likely to be anxious when a child has frequent illnesses than when a correct diagnosis of asthma is given and suitable treatment deals with the problems and reduces time spent off school.

Diagnosis

Asthma is diagnosed in children by breathing tests, or by provoking symptoms with some simple exercise. In young children any testing using instruments such as peak flow meters is very difficult and it may be necessary for the doctor to make the diagnosis on the medical history and the child's response to treatment. Night-time symptoms are common in asthma, particularly in children, and coughing rather than wheezing may be the main feature.

Outlook

Parents are naturally very keen to know whether their child will grow out of asthma. This question has been discussed on p. 26. To some extent it depends on the severity of the asthma. Children with mild intermittent asthma have a 50% chance of losing all their wheezing problems as adults but this is much less likely for those with continuous, severe symptoms. Boys have a better outlook than girls, although they are twice as likely to have asthma in the first place. Even if asthma disappears in teenage years there is still a chance that it will return later. The underlying tendency of the airways to be irritable seems to remain and may produce problems again when a particular stimulus to the lungs is met.

Right treatment improves outlook

It seems that the long term outlook for asthma is better if the condition is well controlled by the right treatment. Many asthmatic children lose a lot of time from school with their attacks. Surveys have shown that if these children are treated in the right way with suitable regular treatment the time they lose from school can often be greatly reduced. It is important, therefore, to aim for good control of the asthma and not to put up with persistent symptoms unnecessarily or just to respond to each attack.

> **Staying well on top of the asthma is important for the short term and long term prospects of the child.**

Treatment

Most earlier chapters on treatment, both drug and non-drug treatment, applies to children as well as to adults but there are some special considerations in children. Allergic factors such as house dust mites, pollens, and family pets tend to be more noticeable with children's asthma than adults'. Avoidance of these allergens is, therefore, more important — as far as this is possible. This will generally mean avoiding household pets and keeping down house dust in the child's bedroom. Cuddly toys can be a good source of house dust mite and should be regularly washed if they are likely to share the child's bed.

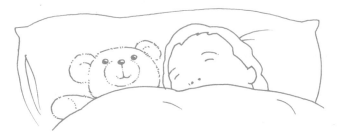

Drug treatment

In general, the treatments used for adult asthma are also those which are most useful for children. There are a few general differences in response, the doses are smaller, and there is the problem of getting the drugs into the airways since it is more difficult to teach very young children to use inhaler devices. Syrup preparations of beta-adrenergic and theophylline bronchodilators are available for children unable to use any sort of inhaler. Theophyllines can be useful for night-time asthma but may cause bowel upsets or vomiting and may perhaps lead to difficulties in concentration and behaviour in children.

In children under 18 months it is difficult to be sure of the diagnosis of asthma. The airways are small at this age and any chest infection may be accompanied by wheezing. Most children who have occasional wheezing at this age do not go on to develop asthma later. When asthma does occur in such young children it also may be difficult to treat. The response to beta-adrenergic drugs such as salbutamol in a nebuliser may be much less impressive than in older children. An anti-cholinergic drug such as ipratropium bromide in a nebuliser may be more effective.

Giving treatment

The metered dose spray inhalers are difficult for young children to use but children over 8 are as good as, or better than, adults with these inhalers. The dry powder inhalers which are available for bronchodilators, corticosteroids and sodium cromoglycate can be used by younger children down to 2 or 3 years old. An alternative is to use a metered dose spray inhaler with some sort of chamber or spacer device to reduce the speed of the spray and to make co-ordination of breath and inhaler use less important. The large globular spacers have been shown to be effective in chronic asthma and in acute attacks of asthma in children. In emergencies it is possible to adapt everyday materials such as polystyrene coffee cups into makeshift spacers to use with inhalers.

Nebulisers can be used by children of all ages although some may dislike the masks and prefer mouthpieces. Broncho-dilators, steroids, and sodium cromoglycate can be given in nebulisers which can be used for regular treatment two to four times each day or for acute attacks. If nebulisers are used for

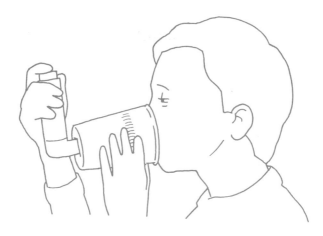

acute attacks it is important to remember that if they are not effective or if they have only a short-lived effect then some other treatment from a general practitioner or in hospital is urgently required.

Growth

Two factors may interfere with growth in asthmatic children. Asthma itself may reduce height but the condition must be severe and continuous to produce this effect. Moderate asthma may delay the onset of puberty. The other factor is corticosteroid treatment, but growth is only affected by prolonged use of oral steroids. Short courses of oral steroids and the use of conventional doses of inhaled steroids do not cause any growth problems. They are important parts of the treatment of asthma and generally are more likely to improve growth by controlling troublesome asthma.

Chest deformities

Prolonged severe asthma may lead to chest deformities but this is uncommon now.

School

Many asthmatic children need to take drugs regularly and to have inhalers available for extra use. It is important that the child's school teachers know of the condition and are informed what to do if there are problems with asthma. Many teachers will need education about the general approach to asthma. They may want to keep children away from games and may be wary of the use of inhalers at school. Parents sometimes need to recruit the help of their family or hospital doctor in developing a sensible plan for an asthmatic child at school.

There was a tendency in the past to send asthmatic children to special schools where their 'weak chests' could be pampered. Some of these schools were at high altitudes where asthma does tend to be better. Improvements in treatment mean that very few asthmatics now require any special school facilities. Residential schools with medical cover do exist for these unusual cases.

> **Most asthmatic children can take part in all physical activities. They should be encouraged to play games at school although they may need to use drugs before playing and to be allowed to ease up in cold or foggy weather.**

Holidays

There are several aspects to consider in arranging holidays for asthmatic children:

- Choose a sensible destination. Many asthmatics are better at the seaside where pollen counts are lower. Alpine mountain resorts have long been known to benefit asthmatics although such improvements rarely last any longer than the holiday.

- Take all the treatment needed. This means a complete supply of regular treatment to cover the holiday and a little extra and any additions to cover an acute attack. It is sensible to go over the details of the acute crisis plan before the holiday to make sure everything is covered. If a nebuliser is used make sure it will work with the local electricity supply. If there is any doubt a simple foot pump nebuliser should be used.
- Find out about the local emergency medical facilities before going, or on arrival. This includes local doctors and hospital facilities, including the times of opening; not all casualty departments function throughout 24 hours.

Adolescence

Fortunately, adolescence is a time when asthma tends to improve. It is also a time when all children can be difficult as they begin to establish their independence. In those with chronic illness this can sometimes take the form of a denial of their problems. It may be difficult to deal with and is best prepared for by educating children about their asthma and involving them in the management of their own condition throughout the earlier years. It is particularly important to discourage smoking in young asthmatics.

Choosing a job

Occupational asthma is considered on p. 49. Asthmatics should generally avoid choosing a job that may cause these problems. They should also try to avoid jobs which will expose them to less specific lung irritants. For instance, it would be best to avoid particularly dusty jobs or those which mean they have to experience frequent changes in air temperature or bad weather conditions.

15 Living with asthma

Asthma is a common condition and its severity varies greatly. A general practitioner will have up to 200 asthmatics among his patients although not all of them will attend with asthmatic symptoms. A typical junior school will have three or four asthmatics in each class and six or seven who have had at least two episodes of wheezing in their short lives.

All these people need to get used to living with their asthma. For some of them this may be a case of taking an occasional puff of their inhaler, perhaps just when they get a cold; for an unfortunate few it may mean never getting rid of their shortness of breath.

Know your asthma

Asthmatic people will get to know the characteristics of their own asthma better than their doctors ever can. It is usually a help to supplement subjective feelings about the way the asthma is behaving with objective measurements with a peak flow meter. This knowledge of the behaviour of the asthma then needs to be applied to the treatment of the condition.

This will mean that adjustments in treatment and searches for causes can be reliably assessed. For instance, if you suspect that reactions to a certain food are contributing to your asthma it is important to judge the effects of withdrawing it from the diet and then, perhaps, reintroducing it. Food sensitivity is not often an important factor in asthma and unless proper assessments are made you may be removing important nutritional elements from your diet unnecessarily. Similarly when you start to use a new inhaler its effect should be monitored. Such monitoring will need careful interpretation since asthma is a variable disease by itself without changes in the treatment.

The modern treatments of asthma are effective and generally very safe. The numerous drugs fall into a few distinct groups (chapters 7, 8 and 9) and it is not at all difficult to understand what your doctor is trying to achieve with the various treatments. This understanding allows an asthmatic to contribute to the treatment.

Asthma societies

Many patients find that they can learn what they need to know about their asthma through their local branch of the Friends of the Asthma Society. The local branches vary in their activity but many of them organise meetings where patients and parents can learn about asthma and bring all their questions to be answered. They can also obtain literature about asthma produced by some of the pharmaceutical societies, the Asthma Society and the British Lung Foundation. Many of these local asthma societies are also involved in the important task of raising money for research into asthma.

The future

There is a great deal of research into asthma, funded by the Asthma Council, the British Lung Foundation, the Medical Research Society and the Chest, Heart and Stroke Association. This research has greatly increased our understanding of the basic underlying mechanisms of asthma. Research is continuing into newer and better treatments. Unfortunately a cure for asthma still seems a long way away but treatment is available to keep most asthmatics well most of the time. In the past our problem has been getting the right treatment to the right patient at the appropriate time. The key to this is education of doctors and of patients to collaborate in the approach. I hope that this book will contribute to this end.

A patient who knows the basic approach is more likely to have the asthma well controlled, less likely to have acute attacks, and less likely to be admitted to hospital.

INDEX